EMERGENCY AND INTENSIVE CARE MEDICINE

SEPTIC SHOCK

RISK FACTORS, MANAGEMENT AND PROGNOSIS

EMERGENCY AND INTENSIVE CARE MEDICINE

Additional books in this series can be found on Nova's website under the Series tab.

Additional e-books in this series can be found on Nova's website under the e-book tab.

EMERGENCY AND INTENSIVE CARE MEDICINE

SEPTIC SHOCK

RISK FACTORS, MANAGEMENT AND PROGNOSIS

BENEDICT GRAVER

EDITOR

New York

Library of Congress Cataloging-in-Publication Data

ISBN: 978-1-63463-916-3
Library of Congress Control Number: 2014960000

Published by Nova Science Publishers, Inc. † New York

Contents

Preface

This book discusses risk factors, management and prognosis of septic shock in individuals.

Chapter I – In a 2013 Healthcare Cost and Utilization Project Statistical Brief by the US Agency for Healthcare Research and Quality, septicemia was ranked as the #1 most expensive national inpatient hospital cost. This ranking comes in spite of substantial advances in the clinical management of sepsis over the past 15 years. While adherence with internationally established sepsis management protocols have demonstrated reduction in mortality and hospital/ICU length of stay, compliance with these protocols remains poor. Contributing factors may be delay in sepsis recognition and protocol implementation. A solution to this barrier is an automated sepsis detection and alert system embedded in the electronic medical record (EMR). In 2013, "alarm hazards" (e.g., excessive alarms, missed alarms, delayed alarms, etc.) was ranked as the #1 health technology hazard by the ECRI (Emergency Care Research Institute). Thus, sepsis surveillance systems must be developed and implemented in the context of alert fatigue, interruption, human error, and information overload. This chapter will describe essential elements in the electronic surveillance system development and implementation processes. Readers will learn about the critical elements of a septic shock detection algorithm and the data needed for each stage of sepsis management, such as early sepsis identification, notification of the clinicians, and tracking treatment processes. The chapter will describe the electronic components for this systems-level control of compliance with internationally established sepsis management protocols. A well-designed severe sepsis surveillance system has the potential to improve protocol compliance and patient outcomes, while reducing healthcare costs.

Chapter II – *Background:* In the scope of analgesia and sedation in intensive care medicine fentanyl was more and more replaced by sufentanil in Europe. Conversely, fentanyl is still more usual worldwide. Furthermore, several advances in the therapy of sepsis were reported. For example, the short-acting ß-blocker esmolol showed positive effects in septic shock. However, for analgesia and sedation in this study a combination of sufentanil and propofol was used. Therefore the question arises whether different results can be expected already because of respectively given analgesics or sedatives. *Methods:* Because the change has been completed in the authors' institution the authors examined the data of their transition period from fentanyl/midazolam (F/M) to sufentanil/midazolam (S/M) retrospectively. As such, 2x12 comparable patients (2x 7 males/5 females, age 50-85 years, 2x3 severe sepsis und 2x9 septic shock) had received either only F/M or only S/M for analgesia and sedation. All accordingly to relevant parameters blind recruited patients were analyzed. The therapeutic aim was (1) the best possible tolerance of intensive care by (2) acceptable compatibility of the used drugs. On the ground of comparable sedation blood pressure, heart rate, laboratory parameters, figures of blood gas analysis and figures of heart rate variability (HRV) were comparatively examined (F/M vs. S/M). For measuring the authors chose the hour of minimal HRV. At this time the CRP as well as the dose of analgesia and sedation was the highest. Furthermore, an explorative correlation analysis was performed. *Results:* Accordingly to the defined therapy target higher analgesic equivalent doses could be given when sufentanil was used ($p<0.001$). Simultaneously, lower midazolam doses had become necessary because of sedative properties of sufentanil by itself ($p=0.008$). Oxygenation could be better performed under S/M (pO_2: $p<0.001$; SO_2: $p=0.005$). Mean blood pressure was less depressed under S/M ($p=0.006$), and the central venous pressure as well ($p=0.015$). On the other hand, heart rate was less elevated under F/M ($p=0.046$). In HRV analysis higher figures of VLF power were found when S/M was used (ln: $p=0.006$). The LF/HF ratio showed vagal predominance in both regimes. However, this was more expressed when F/M was given (0.15 vs. 0.25, $p=0.014$). Further higher values in S/M use were: serum glucose ($p=0.01$), insulin application ($p=0.002$), and body temperature ($p=0.015$). Mortality under infusion or during overhang amounts to 50% in F/M and to 8 % in S/M ($p=0.025$). *Correlation analysis:* A clear inverse connection between heart rate and HRV was found overall: vagal determined parameters ($p\leq0.001$) more than global parameters ($p<0.03$). By contrast, only in F/M use (not in S/M use) the authors found significant associations between metabolic values in the sense of an energetically inefficient anaerobic metabolism: serum glucose vs. serum lactate (r_P=0.745; p=0.005) and pCO_2 vs. pO_2/serum glucose (r_S=0.713; p=0.009). Remarkably, similar coherences that can rather be interpreted as centrally induced dynamic adaptations were only seen when S was used (and not when F/M was used): serum glucose vs. LF/HF ratio (r_P=0.758; p=0.004), systolic blood pressure vs. lnVLF (r_P=0.736; p=0.006), pO_2/FiO_2 vs. lnVLF (r_P=0.705; p=0.01), body temperature vs. SDNN (r_P=–0.703; p=0.011) and SO_2 vs. lnTotal Power (r_P=0.666; p=0.018). Conclusion: The figures from correlation analysis gave hints that the central autonomic regulation will be better preserved by sufentanil/midazolam than by fentanyl/midazolam. The different mortality can be thoroughly explained by the found discrepancies in that period of time when a direct opioid influence is to suppose. As such, the investigation shows that different concepts of analgesia and sedation may have important influences on risk estimating, on therapy management and on prognosis overall. Statements without specification should be re-questioned.

Chapter III – Endothelial cells are essential elements for vascular homeostasis. Their functions are modulated by several molecules, including angiogenesis related factors. The latter are not solely involved in physiological processes such as endothelium maturation and survival, and angiogenesis -a complex process where a new blood vessel is formed from a preexisting one-, but also in pathological conditions, including tumor growth, metastasis and sepsis. Particularly, in severe sepsis the pro-inflammatory state leads to an impairment caused by several mechanisms, resulting into endothelial dysfunction. Angiogenesis-related factors have a pivotal role in the pathophysiological cascade giving rise to this condition, as these molecules contribute to the development of increased capillary permeability, vasoplegia and pro-coagulant and pro-inflammatory states, which could culminate on a septic shock. Recent clinical studies have shown a correlation between the imbalance of the angiogenic growth factors -affecting mainly the angiopoietins and vascular endothelial growth factor pathways- and the poor outcome of patients enduring severe sepsis and septic shock. Different therapies involving the favorable regulation of these angiogenic factors have shown beneficial effects in the pathological events observed in severe sepsis, such as microcirculatory impairment, cardiac fibrosis and hypertrophy, progression towards septic shock and mortality. Therefore, angiogenic growth factors represent a novel prognostic tool in severe sepsis and septic shock. Moreover, these data suggest that angiogenic pathways represent a therapeutic target for future interventions. The design of clinical trials aimed to evaluate the efficacy and safety of anti-angiogenic agents in septic patients is mandatory.

Chapter IV – *Background and Objective*: Accurate differential diagnosis between sepsis and other, non-infectious, causes of systemic inflammatory response syndrome (SIRS) is crucial for timely intervention and survival; however, no single biomarker can confirm pathogen presence in such patients. In this context, the authors assessed Triggered Receptor Expressed on Myelocytes-1 (TREM-1, soluble and membrane-bound forms), a molecule known to propagate systemic inflammation, in regard to its diagnostic value. *Patients and Methods:* Seventy patients were enrolled in total. Group A consisted of 37 adult patients with sepsis, mean age 69.7±15.2 years, diagnosed according to the 2011 Sepsis International Conference criteria (10 with severe sepsis/septic shock and 27 without any organ damage). Group B included 16 patients with systemic autoimmune inflammation (non-infectious SIRS), 8 of them with active rheumatoid arthritis (RA, mean age 65±21 years, Disease Activity Score=4.8±0.8) and 8 with active systemic lupus erythematosus (SLE, mean age 45±5 years, SLE Disease Activity Index=8±2). Group C consisted of 17 healthy individuals for establishing a reference point. Traditional biomarkers, such as C-reactive protein (CRP) and procalcitonin (PCT) were available in the majority of patients. TREM-1 expression on CD14+ monocytes was assessed with flow-cytometry whereas soluble TREM-1 was measured with enzyme-linked immunosorbent assay (ELISA). Statistical analysis was performed with Mann-Whitney U test; $p<0.05$ was considered significant. *Results:* TREM-1 expression on CD14+ macrophages was significantly enhanced in septic patients (50.19±15.79%) in comparison to autoimmune patients (28.2±14%, $p<0.05$) and healthy controls (16.2±10%, $p<0.05$). Likewise, soluble TREM-1 levels were significantly higher in group A (124.6±36.1pg/ml) than group B (43.6±17.4pg/ml, $p<0.05$) and healthy individuals (5±3.3pg/ml, $p<0.05$). Of note, both membrane-bound and soluble TREM-1 did not differ significantly between patients with severe sepsis/septic shock and those without any overt organ damage. *Conclusion:* Patients with sepsis and severe sepsis/septic shock have significantly higher levels of the membrane-bound and soluble forms of TREM-1 compared to active autoimmune patients and healthy individuals. TREM-1 may accurately discriminate infectious from non-infectious SIRS causes.

Chapter V – Multicellular organisms detect danger signals from tissue injury through pattern recognition receptors. These signals serve to initiate the appropriate immune responses that will lead to timely removal of its causative source to prevent further tissue damage. These danger signals, collectively known as damage associated molecular patterns (DAMPs), can be divided into exogenous pathogen associated molecular patterns and endogenous alarmins.

In health, DAMPs work in an orchestrated appropriate manner leading to the clearance of the insult. Dysregulation of DAMPs in disease state can lead to an inappropriate systemic inflammatory response syndrome. Here, we review high mobility group box 1 (HMGB1), a DAMP of significant relevance to the continual propagation of sepsis-induced inflammation. HMGB1, a ubiquitous nuclear protein, released after infection, tissue injury and cell death has been identified as a key late mediator of sepsis-related death in murine models. Unlike early inflammatory mediators where biological pathways have already been activated upon diagnosis of sepsis, HMGB1's delayed role potentially opens a therapeutic window to antagonize its effects. HMGB1's known biological functions and mechanism in which it mediates inflammation, clinical relevance as revealed in human sepsis cohorts and current novel experimental therapeutic intervention are discussed in this review.

In: Septic Shock
Editor: Benedict Graver

ISBN: 978-1-63463-916-3

Chapter I

Septic Shock Electronic Surveillance*

Andrew M. Harrison[1], John G. Park[2] and Vitaly Herasevich[3#]

[1]Medical Scientist Training Program,
Mayo Clinic, Rochester, MN, US
[2]Department of Medicine, Division of Pulmonology and Critical Care Medicine, Mayo Clinic, Rochester MN, US
[3]Department of Anesthesiology, Division of Critical Care,
Mayo Clinic, Rochester, MN, US

Abstract

In a 2013 Healthcare Cost and Utilization Project Statistical Brief by the US Agency for Healthcare Research and Quality, septicemia was ranked as the #1 most expensive national inpatient hospital cost. This ranking comes in spite of substantial advances in the clinical management of sepsis over the past 15 years. While adherence with internationally established sepsis management protocols have demonstrated reduction in

---

* This work was performed at Mayo Clinic in Rochester, MN

Corresponding author: Vitaly Herasevich, Department of Anesthesiology, Mayo Clinic, 200 First Street SW, Rochester, MN 55905, E-Mail: herasevich.vitaly@mayo.edu, Phone: 507-255-9814; Fax: 507-255-4267

mortality and hospital/ICU length of stay, compliance with these protocols remains poor. Contributing factors may be delay in sepsis recognition and protocol implementation. A solution to this barrier is an automated sepsis detection and alert system embedded in the electronic medical record (EMR). In 2013, "alarm hazards" (e.g., excessive alarms, missed alarms, delayed alarms, etc.) was ranked as the #1 health technology hazard by the ECRI (Emergency Care Research Institute). Thus, sepsis surveillance systems must be developed and implemented in the context of alert fatigue, interruption, human error, and information overload. This chapter will describe essential elements in the electronic surveillance system development and implementation processes. Readers will learn about the critical elements of a septic shock detection algorithm and the data needed for each stage of sepsis management, such as early sepsis identification, notification of the clinicians, and tracking treatment processes. The chapter will describe the electronic components for this systems-level control of compliance with internationally established sepsis management protocols. A well-designed severe sepsis surveillance system has the potential to improve protocol compliance and patient outcomes, while reducing healthcare costs.

Detection of Sepsis: Historical Perspective and Current Status (Non-Computerized)

One of the earliest and most crucial steps in sepsis management was the standardization of sepsis and systemic inflammatory response syndrome (SIRS) definitions in August 1991 at a Consensus Conference between the American College of Chest Physicians (ACCP) and the Society of Critical Care Medicine (SCCM) [1]. The standardization of these clinical and physiological biomarkers allowed for early studies of the epidemiology of both sepsis and SIRS [2]. Prior to this, potential molecular biomarkers of sepsis, such as C-reactive protein (CRP), had been identified [3, 4]. In 1993, the first major report of an association between infection, sepsis, and high serum procalcitonin was published [5]. To date, hundreds of additional molecular biomarkers have been examined as potential diagnostic markers for sepsis detection [6]. Some of these molecular biomarkers—such as procalcitonin and CRP—seem to have limited utility in sepsis prognosis. However, none have been validated as diagnostic molecular biomarkers for sepsis detection. The cost-effectiveness of these molecular biomarkers is unclear [7, 8].

In one recent model of hypothetical patients with community-acquired pneumonia, procalcitonin protocol seemed to add $10 – 54 per patient to the cost of care compared to usual care [9].

For the past decade, a study by Martin et al. served as the reference for the epidemiology of sepsis in the United States [10]. A more recent large scale study of severe sepsis and septic shock in Australia and New Zealand demonstrated a significant decrease in mortality between the year 2000 to 2012 [11]. The US Agency for Healthcare Research and Quality (AHRQ) released a Statistical Brief calculating the aggregate cost of septicemia in the US to be $20.3 billion or 5.2% of the total aggregate cost for all hospitalizations [12]. Thus, septicemia is the most expensive inpatient condition to treat, outranking osteoarthritis (#2), complication of device, implant or graft (#3), acute myocardial infarction (#5), and cancer (did not make top 20).

As a result of collaborative work between SCCM and ACCP, consensus definitions for sepsis, severe sepsis, and septic shock have existed for over 20 years [1] with two major revisions [13, 14]. A landmark advancement in sepsis management occurred a decade later with the publication of early goal-directed therapy (EGDT) for the treatment of severe sepsis and septic shock [15]. In this single center research study, early identification and aggressive management of severe sepsis and septic shock in the emergency department (ED) was shown to significantly improve patient outcomes, including mortality. Soon thereafter, the US SCCM and the European Society of Intensive Care Medicine formed the Surviving Sepsis Campaign (SSC) to improve the care of these patients and to improve outcomes. At that time, the goal was to reduce worldwide mortality from severe sepsis and septic shock by 25% in 5 years [16]. This resulted in the publication of the first SSC guidelines for the management of severe sepsis and septic shock in 2004 [17].

With firmly established definitions and guidelines, a rationale exists for the use of computerized sepsis detection systems. At the turn of the century, early hospital alert systems were developed and validated for clinical trial enrollment purposes [18-20]. Likewise, the concept of a critical "golden hour" in the management of acute myocardial infarction and other traumas concurrently gained traction [21-23]. If similar critical hours exist in the management of severe sepsis and septic shock, it should be possible to detect and alert providers to these conditions to reduce response time in the hospital.

Computerized Attempts of Sepsis Detection

The introduction of computers into the hospital and ICU settings is still relatively recent. With the invention of the transistor in the 1940s (Nobel Prize in 1956), discussions of crude hospital EMR systems can be found dating back to the 1960s [24]. Rigorous study of the effect of early EMR systems on hospital practice began in the 1980s [25-27] and in ICU-specific settings a decade later [28-30]. However, due to lack of standardization of sepsis treatment protocols, development of early electronic sepsis surveillance systems did not begin until the 2000s.

In part due to the lack of computerized sepsis detection systems, many challenges hindered a sensitive sepsis detection system. Historically, the basic protocol for management of severe sepsis and septic shock was the administration of appropriate antibiotics, intravenous fluids, and advanced support (such as mechanical ventilation, vasopressors, and dialysis) when necessary [31]. However, the need for better sepsis clinical trials was recognized [32, 33]. Unfortunately, computerized sepsis detection systems could not be refined until standardized sepsis treatment protocols were developed. After the publication of the first SSC guidelines for the management of severe sepsis and septic shock, effectively standardizing sepsis treatment protocols, interest in computerized sepsis detection and alert systems increased dramatically. The current guideline for the diagnosis of sepsis divides the needed data into six clinical categories: general, inflammatory, hemodynamic, organ dysfunction, tissue perfusion, and severe sepsis-specific variables (Table 1). Early prospective electronic sepsis surveillance system studies focused on detection of sepsis, severe sepsis, and/or septic shock in non-ED/ICU settings, ED, and ICU settings [34-36]. These studies provided significant insight into the challenges of automated sepsis detection and alert, but failed to show significant improvement in clinical outcomes upon implementation of these systems. A large single center trial of an automated sepsis detection and alert system (based on modified SIRS criteria) also failed to show significant improvement in clinical outcomes [37]. However, this detection system's positive predictive value was only 41%, which may explain the lack of outcomes improvement. One of the earliest sepsis detection systems, termed the septic shock sniffer, was originally developed and validated at Mayo Clinic to enroll patients with septic shock into a time sensitive clinical trial in the critical care setting [20, 38].

Table 1. Data needs for a severe sepsis and septic shock electronic surveillance system based on current 2012 SSC international guidelines for management of severe sepsis and septic shock

Domain	Value	Rationale	Source in EMR
Age, Gender, Height & weight	any	Demographics implications	Demographics
Suspicion of infection	Presence of any culture order	Systemic infection (sign of sepsis)	Microbiology orders
Heart rate	> 90	SIRS criteria (sign of sepsis)	Monitored data
Respiratory rate	> 20	SIRS criteria (sign of sepsis)	Monitored data
Temperature	> 38 or < 36	SIRS criteria (sign of sepsis)	Monitored data
White blood count	> 12 or < 4	SIRS criteria (sign of sepsis)	Laboratory tests
Lactate	≥ 4.0	Sign of hypoperfusion (severe sepsis)	Laboratory tests
Systolic Blood Pressure	< 90	Sign of hypotension (severe sepsis)	Monitored data
Mean Arterial Pressure	< 70	Sign of hypotension (severe sepsis)	Monitored data
Bilirubin	> 4.0	Sign of organ dysfunction (severe sepsis)	Laboratory tests
Platelets	< 100k	Sign of organ dysfunction (severe sepsis)	Laboratory tests
INR	> 1.5	Sign of organ dysfunction (severe sepsis)	Laboratory tests
Mechanical Ventilation	Any use	Sign of organ dysfunction (severe sepsis)	Monitored data
PaO2/FiO2	< 300	Sign of organ dysfunction (severe sepsis)	Monitored data
GCS score	< 15	Sign of hypoperfusion (severe sepsis)	Nursing flow sheets
Creatinine Increase	> 0.5	Sign of organ dysfunction (severe sepsis)	Laboratory tests
Urine Output	< 0.5 mL/kg/hour for > 2 hours	Sign of organ dysfunction (severe sepsis)	Fluids in and out
Fluid resistant hypotension	SBP < 90 after sufficient fluid bolus	Sign of septic shock	Fluids in and out
Vasopressors	Any use	Sign of septic shock	Medications

The creation of this septic shock sniffer was possible due to the existence of a Multidisciplinary Epidemiology and Translational Research in Intensive Care (METRIC) Data Mart, which aggregates necessary components of patient's data that are usually stored in independent databases [39]. Briefly, this near real-time database copies and stores all ICU data on all ICU patients at Mayo Clinic. This data includes demographics, monitored data (vital signs, ventilator settings, etc.), laboratory tests, transfusions, microbiology, radiology, medications, physician notes, nursing flow sheets, respiratory data, and fluid balance data. Further validated methodology has been developed at Mayo Clinic to improve the severe sepsis and septic shock sniffer for clinical use in the ICU setting [40].

Limitations and Challenges of Early Computerized Systems

The early electronic sepsis surveillance systems described above suffered from a variety of limitations. In particular, many of these earlier studies placed more emphasis on algorithm development than attention to factors such as alert fatigue [41], interruption [42], human error [43], and information overload [44, 45]. Without careful consideration of these implementation factors, even a "perfect" sepsis detection and alert algorithm will fail to improve clinically significant outcomes, such as mortality and hospital/ICU length of stay. An inherent limitation of these earlier studies is also their single center design. Even the best single center, prospective study will potentially suffer from a variety of common epidemiologic biases and/or confounders [46]. These early electronic sepsis surveillance systems also needed to overcome numerous informatics challenges. Although less than one decade old, the timing of these studies overlaps with the rise of the concept and recognition of "big data" (i.e., large and complex sets of data that may be difficult to process and analyze using traditional systems). In less than a decade, the concept of big data has permeated fields ranging from biomedical research [47] to business/finance [48, 49] to healthcare and clinical research [50]. However, without sufficiently complex electronic infrastructure and personnel support, the same limitations and challenges outlined as implementation factors above are only amplified in clinical studies requiring use of big data.

Since these early electronic sepsis surveillance studies, many more single center studies have been conducted [51-56]. The scope of each of these studies varies significantly—study design, hospital setting, and number of patients—while suffering from the single center limitations and challenges outlined above. However, with sufficient experience systemic reviews of this topic are being published [57]. Likewise, a large multicenter/international study was recently conducted using SSC data [58] to produce a "sepsis severity score" [59]. This study was designed primarily for prognostication with population-level case mix adjustments, as opposed to patient-level, diagnostics purposes. Nonetheless, this study represents a landmark in the field of sepsis detection and alert systems.

Elements of an Advanced Computerized System

A "perfect" electronic sepsis surveillance system will not have close to the 99% sensitivity and specificity of FDA-approved rapid HIV tests [60]. This is due to differences in the complexity and nature of these tasks. When the ability of the SIRS criteria (an important element of any sepsis detection algorithm) to identify infection is compared against both clinical and microbiological gold standards; sensitivity, specificity, positive predictive value, and negative predictive value are all relatively poor [61]. For example, the sensitivity of the SIRS criteria against both gold standards (defined as dismissal diagnosis of sepsis or evidence of microbiological growth from any culture site) was 69%, while the specificity against these gold standards was 35% and 32%, respectively. Likewise, it is important to recognize that the accuracy of any test is dependent not only on the test characteristics, but also the prevalence of disease, among other factors [62]. Nonetheless, a perfect electronic sepsis surveillance system should achieve several goals.

First, an ideal electronic sepsis surveillance system should only generate actionable alerts in the context of alert fatigue, interruption, human error, and information overload. For example, electronic sepsis surveillance systems should not generate alerts for suspicion of infection or presence of SIRS criteria in isolation. This is because many patients in the critical care setting have suspicion of an infection due to SIRS criteria but may not have sepsis (e.g., drug fever or deep vein thrombosis). Furthermore, only a fraction of septic patients progress to severe sepsis (sepsis with the presence of organ dysfunction) or septic shock. In the absence of significant comorbidities, it is only at the level of severe sepsis that mortality due to sepsis rises significantly [63]. Interestingly, it is also unclear if meaningful alerts could be generated in the context of septic shock. Although mortality in this extremely time-sensitive circumstance is even higher than severe sepsis, EMR-based detection of sepsis relies on existing EMR data. In other words, the presence of fluid resistant hypotension and/or the use of vasopressors (elements of the definition of septic shock) imply the presence of septic shock has already been identified by providers and action has been taken. Alerts in these contexts would potentially lead to alert fatigue, interruption, human error, and information overload. Thus, from the perspective of the clinical continuum from sepsis to septic shock, one of the clearest targets for actionable alerts is the critical golden hours during the progression from severe sepsis to septic shock. Adherence to existing, international SSC guidelines for severe sepsis and septic shock are known to significantly reduce mortality [58]. However, compliance with these guidelines is poor. There is frequently a delay between the generation of lab values, such as biomarkers of organ dysfunction, and clinician awareness of these values. Thus, preventing the progression of severe sepsis to septic shock is one mechanism to generate actionable sepsis alerts to reduce mortality in the critical care setting. The current SSC guidelines [14] are highly detailed, but contain a simplified set of two "bundles". The first bundle is comprised of a set of 4 elements to be completed within 3 hours upon suspicion and/or diagnosis of sepsis, while the second bundle is comprised of 3 elements to be completed within 6 hours. However, it should be noted that these bundle elements are not all mutually exclusive and can form a feedback loop. For example, it is expected that 30 mL/kg of crystalloid fluids will be administered within 3 hours for hypotension or elevated lactate. However, it is also expected that vasopressors will be administered within 6 hours if hypotension is not adequately reversed with fluids. Should hypotension persist (evidence of septic shock), it is thus possible to cycle between fluid administration and vasopressor use for periods of time much greater than 6 hours. Similarly, the first element of the 3-hour bundle is lactate measurement. However, both persistent hypotension and the third element of the 6-hour bundle (re-measure lactate if initial lactate was elevated) can result in feedback loop of repeated lactate measurements for an indefinite period of time. Secondly, an ideal electronic sepsis surveillance system must do more than detect sepsis. Once severe sepsis and/or septic shock have been identified, timely and appropriate response according to SSC guidelines remains crucial for positive patient outcomes [64]. Thus, identification of failure to comply with these guidelines in a timely and appropriate manner is another potential mechanism for actionable sepsis alerts. Additionally, alerts need to be sent to the correct provider using the correction mechanism of alert delivery. This subject is particularly important in the context of alert hazards and has been studied in the context of the development of monitoring and alert systems for geriatric patients in the home setting [65, 66]. However, relatively limited investigation into methods of alert delivery to these patients' providers in the hospital setting has been performed [67]. Furthermore, this subject has been explored even less in the critical care setting [68, 69]. As the age of the average ICU patient is around 65 years and studies in the critical care setting are lacking [70], this example of geriatric patients is particularly relevant to highlight the specific need to perform systematic investigation of alert processes in the critical care/ICU setting. Specifically, most of the automated sepsis detection and alert systems previously referenced provided alerts to attending physicians using text paging as the mechanism of alert delivery. However, the questions of who should be the recipient of urgent and/or non-urgent alerts (attending physicians, residents/fellows, NPs/PAs, RNs, etc.) and how these alerts should be delivered—text paging, EMR-based messaging, email, or smartphone [71]—remain unresolved.

What EMR Data Is Needed?

To achieve the goals for an ideal electronic sepsis surveillance system, specific data requirements are necessary. The current 2012 SSC international guidelines for management of severe sepsis and septic shock provide a good starting point for these requirements [14]. These specific data requirements include a variety of variables/domains as diagnostic criteria for sepsis, as well as cutoff values for quantitative variables/domains, all of which can be extracted from the EMR. Conceptually, some of these variables/domains have varying degrees of usefulness along the sepsis "spectrum": suspicion of infection *or* SIRS, sepsis (suspicion of infection *and* SIRS), severe sepsis, or septic shock. It should be noted that not all of the numerous data elements listed in the current SSC guidelines are necessary to create an ideal electronic sepsis surveillance system. One example is hyperglycemia in the absence of diabetes. Although there are other important reasons to prevent hyperglycemia in critically ill patients, this value can change rapidly and is not required for the diagnosis of sepsis, severe sepsis, or septic shock. As glycemic state can change rapidly, this limits the usefulness of this marker for quick detection of sepsis. Alternatively, decreased urine output for more than two hours despite adequate fluid resuscitation is a marker of organ/renal dysfunction (severe sepsis). However, the many hours potentially required to make this observation also limits the usefulness of this marker for timely detection of severe sepsis. It is therefore necessary to build an electronic sepsis surveillance system that includes other markers of organ dysfunction/severe sepsis, such as increased creatinine, increased bilirubin, and decreased platelet count. However, this implies that the detection algorithm must include the ability to detect changes in these variables rather the absolute values. Combined, carefully and correctly selected data from the EMR must be used to create the ideal system. In addition to previously discussed human-centric limitations and challenges—such as alert fatigue, interruption, human error, and information overload—there are also human-independent limitations to an ideal electronic sepsis surveillance system. In the context of "big data", the need for real-time, accurate data at the bedside ("point of care") is a crucial challenge. It is already known that the positive effect of point of care computer reminders on processes and outcomes of care in the hospital setting is limited (72). While some of this may be due to human-dependent factors, this does not entirely explain this observation. For example, there are uncertainties in the EMR systems, such as whether most of the variables/domains listed in Table 1 were ordered, if the timestamps represent time the test was ordered or the time the results were completed, and what the lag-time is in reporting new data. In a healthcare center of any size, complete data availability and interoperability of any electronic sepsis surveillance system may not exist across the ICU, ED, OR, and/or hospital floors (with or without telemetry). This can be due to lack of backend electronic infrastructure to support an electronic sepsis surveillance system in the context of an existing EMR system. The complexity of this problem is compounded when considering a multisite healthcare system, as data availability and interoperability across physical locations may be severely limited.

Workflow Changes, Educational Challenges, and Implementation

Knowledge is only the first step in the successful implementation of any complex technical system, medical or otherwise, which significantly modifies or alters an existing, complex system. In this case, the SSC has provided the knowledge necessary to manage severe sepsis and septic shock. Thus, clinical knowledge of sepsis is not the primary barrier for implementation of an electronic sepsis surveillance system in the ICU and other hospital settings. Initial barriers include workflow and education changes. Even an ideal electronic sepsis surveillance system will not be accepted by clinicians (attending physicians, residents/fellows, NPs/PAs, RNs, etc.) unless the system is first introduced without substantially changing the existing workflow process for sepsis management. In the case of Mayo Clinic, this involved first creating METRIC Data Mart (a near real-time, EMR-independent information database), as well as the Ambient Warning and Response Evaluation (AWARE) system, an ICU-specific EMR viewer, for use as a platform in the critical care setting, on top of the existing EMR system [73]. Once a system has been introduced into the existing workflow, implementation changes must occur through educational interventions. The first steps involve active training sessions and prominently displayed poster-style reminders in the critical care setting. After these educational interventions and initial implementation, continued implementation efforts are required. This entails clear mechanisms and response to both unstructured (feedback button) and structured data (survey) for both the critical care and other monitored settings [74]. Each of these components of the implementation process, including post-marketing surveillance, is crucial for the success of an ideal sepsis electronic surveillance algorithm [75]. Essentially, implementation of an electronic sepsis surveillance system is similar to implementation of new therapeutics, medical devices, and even direct-to-consumer advertising.

Perspectives

After the publication of the first set of SSC guidelines for management of severe sepsis and septic shock in 2004 [17], one issue was identified with these guidelines: the lack of a clear, linear, bulleted management protocol to accompany the 16-page document [76]. As a result, the first SSC "bundles" for sepsis management were published the following year [16]. More importantly, this was a realization that lengthy, elaborate guidelines were not successfully implemented in the absence of a straightforward and human-interpretable summary of these processes in diagram format. From that point, although the second [13] and third (current) [13, 14] editions of the SSC guidelines approximately doubled and tripled in size with respect to the initial guidelines, the SSC "bundles" were also updated and prominently incorporated into both the SSC guideline document and website.

Unfortunately, although the SSC bundles continue to mature, both the current SSC bundles and guidelines are *not* machine-readable/interpretable. For example, the fourth component of the 3-hour SSC bundle is to administer 30 mL/kg crystalloid for hypotension. However, for a computer to calculate the success or failure of completion of this intervention, several variables are required within this 3-hour window: blood pressure readings, fluid administration, and weight. Although blood pressure readings may be easily obtained, tracking fluid administration (specifically, bolus-only) is more complex. Additionally, in regard to EMR-interoperability, what if fluids are administered first in the ED setting, but then continued in the ICU setting? Does an electronic sepsis surveillance system have the capacity to track and understand fluid-bolus continuity across clinical departments? What if 30 mL/kg crystalloid for hypotension is achieved in 3.1 hours? In other words, what might be considered as a success by a clinician (aka human) would be considered a failure by the computer (aka machine). Even worse, a patient's weight might not be entered during the first 3 hours. In the absence of a weight to calculate the required fluid bolus, a computer would be forced to register all fluid boluses as failures. From a clinical perspective, this point may seem irrelevant, as many patient weights can be estimated. One solution is to collect all patient weights for the specific purpose of satisfying the algorithm. However, this concept is in opposition to earlier concepts of the implementation process: the machine should serve the clinician and not vice versa. Another solution is to expand the algorithm's ability to search for weights prior to 3 hours. But how far in advance of 3 hours and who decides this important cutoff value? Similar challenges related to this issue are also present in other elements of both the 3 and 6-hour SSC bundles.

Ultimately, as the rise of evidence-based medicine and education continues [77, 78], increased emphasis will be placed on adherence to "best practice" protocols, such as the SSC guidelines. However, the future of evidence-based medicine and education hinges on the question of the need/desire for clinicians to interpret free-text protocols versus reliance on potentially "black box" machine algorithms. For this shift to electronic surveillance systems to occur, best practice protocols must shift from clinical interpretation to computer/coding-friendly language. Otherwise, as the number and complexity of best practice protocols continues to expand, the benefits of human interpretable algorithms in evidence-based medicine will slowly be lost to the inability to translate these algorithms into electronic systems that can handle volumes of data, which otherwise lead to alert fatigue, interruption, human error, and information overload. Thus, clinicians must eventually reassess the place for and implications of electronic surveillance systems in modern medicine.

It is also necessary to implement an electronic sepsis surveillance system using the correct delivery platform. One option is to implement these systems through existing commercial [79], open access [80], and/or custom EMR platforms. Another option is to use a custom delivery platform in parallel with an existing EMR system. For example, Mayo Clinic is implementing its electronic sepsis surveillance system in the critical care setting through AWARE, the ICU-specific patient viewer developed at Mayo Clinic and in use in routine clinical practice across its Minnesota, Arizona, and Florida locations, which have different core EMRs [81, 82]. Regardless of the delivery platform, an electronic sepsis surveillance system should interact synergistically with other electronic systems to reduce the alert hazards described above.

Future Algorithm Improvements for Electronic Surveillance

In the recent US multicenter ProCESS Trial, early-goal directed therapy (EGDT) was demonstrated to not significantly differ from "protocol-based standard therapy" or the current standard of care [83]. These results are supported by another recent multicenter trial in Australia and New Zealand (ARISE), comparing EGDT to "usual care" [84]. Taken together, these results indicate the success of sepsis diagnosis and management efforts over the past 20+ years. These results further indicate that some elements of the SSC bundle may not be essential in the management of septic patients.

It is also important to recognize the widespread scope of interest in improving sepsis outcomes. One current example not highlighted in this chapter is nursing. For many decades, the academic nursing community has published sepsis outcomes in nursing journals, in parallel with general medical journals [85]. Another example is veterinary medicine. In addition to sepsis outcomes, the veterinary literature routinely publishes interesting sepsis case reports on par or more interesting than those published in the general (human) medical journals [86]. In the area of dental hygiene, a recent randomized clinical trial showed that routine dental care/treatment of critically ill patients in the ICU setting significantly reduces lower respiratory tract infections [87]. These studies represent examples of many diverse interests within the healthcare community devoted to improving sepsis outcomes now and in the future.

In order to develop a truly intelligent electronic sepsis surveillance system, it is necessary to consider more factors that have not yet been described in detail in this chapter, such as workflow analysis, ambience, and feedback [88]. In particular, existing electronic sepsis surveillance systems have focused specifically on sepsis detection and alert. However, such systems can be improved through implementation of automated detection and alert systems in the specific context of failure to rescue and treat sepsis in a timely and appropriate manner after diagnosis, which has already been shown to reduce mortality [58, 64]. As will be described below, failure to rescue and treat sepsis differs from failure to recognize sepsis in that this component of electronic sepsis surveillance focuses on response after the detection of sepsis. These concepts have not been explored in existing electronic sepsis surveillance systems.

In addition to the data needed and the implementation process, it is necessary to consider additional factors to develop a truly intelligent electronic sepsis surveillance system. One of these factors is the concept of "failure to rescue" (Figure 1). The US AHRQ (Agency for Healthcare Research and Quality) Patient Safety Network defines failure to rescue as "shorthand for failure to rescue (i.e., prevent a clinically important deterioration, such as death or permanent disability) from a complication of an underlying illness (e.g., cardiac arrest in a patient with acute myocardial infarction) or a complication of medical care (e.g., major hemorrhage after thrombolysis for acute myocardial infarction). Failure to rescue thus provides a measure of the degree to which providers responded to adverse occurrences (e.g., hospital-acquired infections, cardiac arrest, or shock) that developed on their watch. It may reflect the quality of monitoring, the effectiveness of actions taken once early complications are recognized, or both." [89]. This concept and term is derived from studies performed by Silber and colleagues over two decades ago in the surgical setting [90, 91]. Over the next decade, they extended these studies into perioperative areas such as anesthesiology [92] and nursing [93]. This concept of failure to rescue was recently applied to perform comparative analysis, at the hospital-wide level, across multiple institutions to assess availability of hospital resources and differences in performance [94]. However, like previous studies, the underlying population of interest was surgical patients. With this recent study in mind, Silber and colleagues are now exploring failure to rescue as a component for standardizing patients for hospital audit/evaluation purposes and cost analysis [95]. However, the concept of failure to rescue outside the perioperative realm, including the ICU setting, remains largely unexplored.

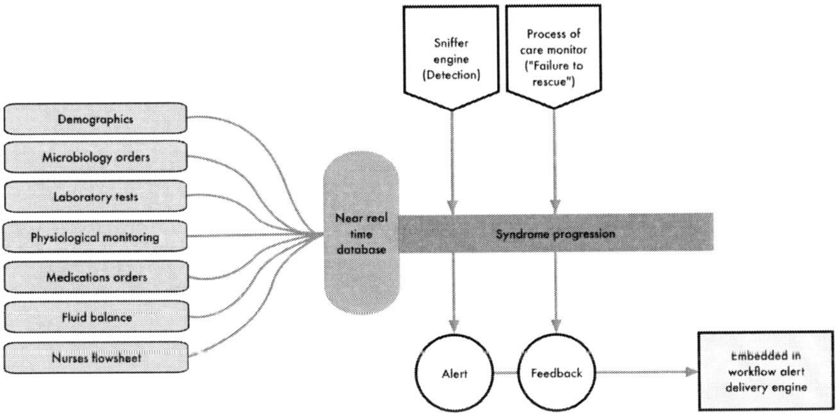

Figure 1. Flow diagram of sepsis management in the context of detection, failure to treat, and failure to rescue alerts, as well as physiologically relevant variables.

An electronic sepsis surveillance system with the capacity to identify failure to rescue and treat sepsis in a timely and appropriate manner after diagnosis—in addition to sepsis detection/recognition—has the potential to intelligently prevent alert fatigue, interruption, human error, and information overload. Along these lines, the methodology for this system has already been retrospectively validated for implementation at Mayo Clinic using an improved severe sepsis and septic shock "sniffer" for clinical use in the ICU setting [40]. Likewise, researchers at Mayo Clinic have already shown that activation of a sepsis response team, in combination with weekly feedback, increases the compliance with processes of care and reduces hospital mortality rate in the setting of septic shock [96]. Thus, future implementation of complex electronic surveillance systems, such as a sepsis sniffer with a failure to rescue component, can only occur in combination with these other mechanisms of diagnosis and management of septic patients.

The final element of future algorithm improvements in the context of electronic surveillance is the human interpretability of these algorithms. Guideline adherence can be improved by combining a refined sepsis alert and detection system with existing electronic infrastructures to further improve sepsis outcomes. The development of the surveillance algorithm for the detection of failure to recognize and treat severe sepsis in the Mayo Clinic study described above made use of recursive data partitioning analysis. This technique is considered to be an advanced modeling and multivariate method, which has been described in detail elsewhere [97]. Briefly, statistical partitioning allows for the division of a data set into a complete, but non-overlapping, collection of components or parts using decision tress. It should be noted that other mathematical modeling approaches for sepsis detection and alert have been developed. For example, one unrelated study made use of a Dynamic Bayesian Networks-based model for early detection of sepsis in the ED setting [98]. Another group used machine learning-based models to develop a decision support system to make clinical predictions for patients with sepsis [99]. Thus, alternative modeling techniques may be applicable to the development of detection and alert systems specific to failure to rescue and treat sepsis.

Human interpretability of algorithms generated by a machine, such as supervised learning techniques (Bayesian networks, neural networks, and ensemble learning), or heuristic optimization techniques is often limited [100]. Thus, with increasing prevalence of complex technologies throughout the hospital setting, clinicians must eventually determine what is and is not an acceptable loss of human interpretability to "black box" algorithms. This will be particularly important if implementation of these algorithms results in improved patient outcomes. Ideally, this equilibrium will evolve in parallel with other improvements in the understanding of both the pathophysiology and clinical management of sepsis.

Bullet Points

(1) Detection of sepsis: historical perspective and current status (non-computerized)

- Consensus conference criteria, early-goal directed therapy, and the Surviving Sepsis Campaign provided the basis for the clinical diagnosis and management of sepsis.

(2) Computerized attempts

- The earliest sepsis detection systems were developed primarily for clinical trial enrollment purposes, while recent, largely retrospective studies have focused on improvement of clinical outcomes in both critically and non-critically ill patients in ICU, ED, and hospital floor settings.

(3) Limitations and challenges of early systems

- In addition to retrospective and algorithmic limitations, a challenge of the above systems has been to address alert fatigue, interruption, human error, and information overload.

(4) Elements of an advanced system.

- An ideal electronic sepsis surveillance system should address all of the above challenges and delivery alerts to the correct providers to improve clinical outcomes, but still will not achieve 100% accuracy.

(5) Data needs

- The hospital EMR-infrastructure must be capable of integrating SSC international guidelines in the context of real-time data availability and interoperability across all relevant hospital settings (ICU, ED, and hospital floors).

(6) Workflow changes, educational changes, and implementation

- Implementation of a "perfect" electronic sepsis surveillance system will fail without the proper workflow and educational interventions to achieve acceptance from clinicians.

(7) Perspectives

- SSC guidelines are readable by humans, but not necessarily computer algorithms, which hampers the development of evidence-based electronic sepsis surveillance systems.

(8) Future algorithm improvements in the context of electronic surveillance

- In addition to detection/recognition, future algorithms must integrate the concepts of failure to rescue and treat sepsis with advanced modeling techniques, which may also result in a decrease in the human interpretability ("black box") of these algorithms.

References

[1] Bone RC, Balk RA, Cerra FB, et al. Definitions for sepsis and organ failure and guidelines for the use of innovative therapies in sepsis. The ACCP/SCCM Consensus Conference Committee. American College of Chest Physicians/Society of Critical Care Medicine. *Chest* 1992;101(6):1644-1655.

[2] Bone RC. Toward an epidemiology and natural history of SIRS (systemic inflammatory response syndrome). *JAMA : the journal of the American Medical Association* 1992;268(24):3452-3455.

[3] Sabel KG, Wadsworth C. C-reactive protein (CRP) in early diagnosis of neonatal septicemia. *Acta Paediatr Scand.* 1979;68(6):825-831.

[4] Sganga G, Siegel JH, Brown G, et al. Reprioritization of hepatic plasma protein release in trauma and sepsis. *Arch. Surg.* 1985;120(2):187-199.

[5] Assicot M, Gendrel D, Carsin H, et al. High serum procalcitonin concentrations in patients with sepsis and infection. *Lancet* 1993;341(8844):515-518.

[6] Pierrakos C, Vincent JL. Sepsis biomarkers: a review. *Critical care* 2010;14(1):R15.

[7] Heyland DK, Johnson AP, Reynolds SC, et al. Procalcitonin for reduced antibiotic exposure in the critical care setting: a systematic review and an economic evaluation. *Crit. Care Med.* 2011;39(7):1792-1799.

[8] Prkno A, Wacker C, Brunkhorst F, et al. Procalcitonin-guided therapy in intensive care unit patients with severe sepsis and septic shock - a systematic review and meta-analysis. *Critical Care* 2013;17(6):R291.

[9] Smith KJ, Wateska A, Nowalk MP, et al. Cost-effectiveness of procalcitonin-guided antibiotic use in community acquired pneumonia. *J. Gen. Intern Med.* 2013;28(9):1157-1164.

[10] Martin GS, Mannino DM, Eaton S, et al. The epidemiology of sepsis in the United States from 1979 through 2000. *N. Engl. J. Med.* 2003;348(16):1546-1554.

[11] Kaukonen KM, Bailey M, Suzuki S, et al. Mortality related to severe sepsis and septic shock among critically ill patients in Australia and New

Zealand, 2000-2012. *JAMA : the journal of the American Medical Association* 2014;311(13):1308-1316.

[12] Torio CM AR. National Inpatient Hospital Costs: The Most Expensive Conditions by Payer, 2011. *HCUP Statistical Brief* 2013;#160.

[13] Dellinger RP, Levy MM, Carlet JM, et al. Surviving Sepsis Campaign: international guidelines for management of severe sepsis and septic shock: 2008. *Crit. Care Med.* 2008;36(1):296-327.

[14] Dellinger RP, Levy MM, Rhodes A, et al. Surviving sepsis campaign: international guidelines for management of severe sepsis and septic shock: 2012. *Crit. Care Med.* 2013;41(2):580-637.

[15] Rivers E, Nguyen B, Havstad S, et al. Early goal-directed therapy in the treatment of severe sepsis and septic shock. *N. Engl. J. Med.* 2001;345(19):1368-1377.

[16] Levy MM, Pronovost PJ, Dellinger RP, et al. Sepsis change bundles: converting guidelines into meaningful change in behavior and clinical outcome. *Crit. Care Med.* 2004;32(11 Suppl):S595-597.

[17] Dellinger RP, Carlet JM, Masur H, et al. Surviving Sepsis Campaign guidelines for management of severe sepsis and septic shock. *Crit. Care Med.* 2004;32(3):858-873.

[18] Thompson DS, Oberteuffer R, Dorman T. Sepsis alert and diagnostic system: integrating clinical systems to enhance study coordinator efficiency. *Comput Inform Nurs* 2003;21(1):22-26; quiz 27-28.

[19] Embi PJ, Jain A, Clark J, et al. Effect of a clinical trial alert system on physician participation in trial recruitment. *Arch. Intern Med.* 2005;165(19):2272-2277.

[20] Herasevich V, Afessa B, Chute CG, et al. Designing and testing computer based screening engine for severe sepsis/septic shock. *AMIA Annu Symp Proc* 2008:966.

[21] Boersma E, Maas AC, Deckers JW, et al. Early thrombolytic treatment in acute myocardial infarction: reappraisal of the golden hour. *Lancet* 1996;348(9030):771-775.

[22] Blow O, Magliore L, Claridge JA, et al. The golden hour and the silver day: detection and correction of occult hypoperfusion within 24 hours improves outcome from major trauma. *J. Trauma* 1999;47(5):964-969.

[23] Lerner EB, Moscati RM. The golden hour: scientific fact or medical "urban legend"? *Acad. Emerg. Med.* 2001;8(7):758-760.

[24] Siegel SJ. Developing an information system for a hospital. *Public Health Rep.* 1968;83(5):359-362.

[25] McDonald CJ, Wilson GA, McCabe GP, Jr. Physician response to computer reminders. *JAMA* 1980;244(14):1579-1581.

[26] McDonald CJ, Hui SL, Smith DM, et al. Reminders to physicians from an introspective computer medical record. A two-year randomized trial. *Annals of internal medicine* 1984;100(1):130-138.

[27] McDonald CJ, Tierney WM. Computer-stored medical records. Their future role in medical practice. *JAMA* 1988;259(23):3433-3440.

[28] Cullen DJ, Sweitzer BJ, Bates DW, et al. Preventable adverse drug events in hospitalized patients: a comparative study of intensive care and general care units. *Crit. Care Med.* 1997;25(8):1289-1297.

[29] Tsien CL, Fackler JC. Poor prognosis for existing monitors in the intensive care unit. *Crit. Care Med.* 1997;25(4):614-619.

[30] Sado AS. Electronic medical record in the intensive care unit. *Crit Care Clin* 1999;15(3):499-522.

[31] Balk RA. Severe sepsis and septic shock. Definitions, epidemiology, and clinical manifestations. *Crit Care Clin* 2000;16(2):179-192.

[32] Sibbald WJ, Vincent JL. Round table conference on clinical trials for the treatment of sepsis. *Crit. Care Med.* 1995;23(2):394-399.

[33] Nasraway SA, Jr. Sepsis research: we must change course. *Crit. Care Med.* 1999;27(2):427-430.

[34] Sawyer AM, Deal EN, Labelle AJ, et al. Implementation of a real-time computerized sepsis alert in nonintensive care unit patients. *Crit. Care Med.* 2011;39(3):469-473.

[35] Nelson JL, Smith BL, Jared JD, et al. Prospective trial of real-time electronic surveillance to expedite early care of severe sepsis. *Ann. Emerg. Med.* 2011;57(5):500-504.

[36] Larosa JA, Ahmad N, Feinberg M, et al. The use of an early alert system to improve compliance with sepsis bundles and to assess impact on mortality. *Crit Care Res Pract* 2012;2012:980369.

[37] Hooper MH, Weavind L, Wheeler AP, et al. Randomized trial of automated, electronic monitoring to facilitate early detection of sepsis in the intensive care unit*. *Crit. Care Med.* 2012;40(7):2096-2101.

[38] Herasevich V, Pieper MS, Pulido J, et al. Enrollment into a time sensitive clinical study in the critical care setting: results from computerized septic shock sniffer implementation. *J. Am. Med. Inform Assoc.* 2011;18(5):639-644.

[39] Herasevich V, Pickering BW, Dong Y, et al. Informatics infrastructure for syndrome surveillance, decision support, reporting, and modeling of critical illness. *Mayo Clin. Proc.* 2010;85(3):247-254.

[40] Harrison AM, Thongprayoon C, Kashyap R, et al. Developing the surveillance algorithm for detection of failure to recognize and treat severe sepsis. *Mayo Clin. Proc.*;In press.

[41] Singh H, Spitzmueller C, Petersen NJ, et al. Information Overload and Missed Test Results in Electronic Health Record-Based Settings. *JAMA Intern Med* 2013:1-3.

[42] Hodgetts HM, Jones DM. Reminders, alerts and pop-ups: The cost of computer-initiated interruptions. In. Beijing; 2007. p. 818-826.

[43] Bates DW, Leape LL, Cullen DJ, et al. Effect of computerized physician order entry and a team intervention on prevention of serious medication errors. JAMA : the journal of the American Medical Association 1998;280(15):1311-1316.

[44] Stokstad E. Information overload hampers biology reforms. *Science* 2001;293(5535):1609.

[45] Dennis C. Information overload. *Nature* 2002;417(6884):14.

[46] Hulley SB, Cummings SR, Browner WS, et al. Designing clinical research: Lippincott Williams & Wilkins; 2006.

[47] Lynch C. Big data: How do your data grow? *Nature* 2008;455(7209):28-29.

[48] Manyika J, Chui M, Brown B, et al. Big data: The next frontier for innovation, competition and productivity.: Technical report, McKinsey Global Institute; 2011.

[49] McAfee A, Brynjolfsson E, Davenport TH, et al. Big Data. The management revolution *Harvard Bus Rev.* 2012;90(10):61-67.

[50] Murdoch TB, Detsky AS. The inevitable application of big data to health care. *JAMA : the journal of the American Medical Association* 2013;309(13):1351-1352.

[51] Brandt BN, Gartner AB, Moncure M, et al. Identifying Severe Sepsis via Electronic Surveillance. *Am. J. Med. Qual.* 2014.

[52] Gur I, Riskin A, Markel G, et al. Pilot Study of a New Mathematical Algorithm for Early Detection of Late-Onset Sepsis in Very Low-Birth-Weight Infants. *Am. J. Perinatol.* 2014.

[53] Hilderink MJ, Roest AA, Hermans M, et al. Predictive accuracy and feasibility of risk stratification scores for 28-day mortality of patients with sepsis in an emergency department. *Eur. J. Emerg. Med.* 2014.

[54] McRee L, Thanavaro JL, Moore K, et al. The impact of an electronic medical record surveillance program on outcomes for patients with sepsis. *Heart Lung* 2014.

[55] Nguyen SQ, Mwakalindile E, Booth JS, et al. Automated electronic medical record sepsis detection in the emergency department. *Peer J.* 2014;2:e343.
[56] Umscheid CA, Betesh J, VanZandbergen C, et al. Development, implementation, and impact of an automated early warning and response system for sepsis. *J. Hosp. Med.* 2014.
[57] Kashiouris M, O'Horo JC, Pickering BW, et al. Diagnostic performance of electronic syndromic surveillance systems in acute care: a systematic review. *Applied Clinical Informatics* 2013;4(2):212-224.
[58] Levy MM, Dellinger RP, Townsend SR, et al. The Surviving Sepsis Campaign: results of an international guideline-based performance improvement program targeting severe sepsis. *Crit. Care Med.* 2010;38(2):367-374.
[59] Osborn TM, Phillips G, Lemeshow S, et al. Sepsis Severity Score: An Internationally Derived Scoring System From the Surviving Sepsis Campaign Database. *Crit. Care Med.* 2014.
[60] Greenwald JL, Burstein GR, Pincus J, et al. A rapid review of rapid HIV antibody tests. *Curr. Infect Dis. Rep.* 2006;8(2):125-131.
[61] Jaimes F, Garces J, Cuervo J, et al. The systemic inflammatory response syndrome (SIRS) to identify infected patients in the emergency room. *Intensive Care Med.* 2003;29(8):1368-1371.
[62] Fischer JE, Bachmann LM, Jaeschke R. A readers' guide to the interpretation of diagnostic test properties: clinical example of sepsis. *Intensive Care Med.* 2003;29(7):1043-1051.
[63] Rezende E, Silva JM, Jr., Isola AM, et al. Epidemiology of severe sepsis in the emergency department and difficulties in the initial assistance. *Clinics* (Sao Paulo) 2008;63(4):457-464.
[64] Levy MM, Rhodes A, Phillips GS, et al. Surviving Sepsis Campaign: Association Between Performance Metrics and Outcomes in a 7.5-Year Study. *Crit. Care Med.* 2014.
[65] Steinman MA, Handler SM, Gurwitz JH, et al. Beyond the prescription: medication monitoring and adverse drug events in older adults. *J. Am. Geriatr Soc.* 2011;59(8):1513-1520.
[66] Tchalla AE, Lachal F, Cardinaud N, et al. Efficacy of simple home-based technologies combined with a monitoring assistive center in decreasing falls in a frail elderly population (results of the Esoppe study). *Arch. Gerontol. Geriatr.* 2012;55(3):683-689.

[67] Loo TS, Davis RB, Lipsitz LA, et al. Electronic medical record reminders and panel management to improve primary care of elderly patients. *Arch. Intern Med.* 2011;171(17):1552-1558.

[68] Wagner MM, Eisenstadt SA, Hogan WR, et al. Preferences of interns and residents for E-mail, paging, or traditional methods for the delivery of different types of clinical information. *Proc. AMIA Symp.* 1998:140-144.

[69] Embi PJ, Jain A, Harris CM. Physicians' perceptions of an electronic health record-based clinical trial alert approach to subject recruitment: a survey. *BMC Med. Inform Decis. Mak.* 2008;8:13.

[70] Seferian EG, Afessa B. Demographic and clinical variation of adult intensive care unit utilization from a geographically defined population. *Crit. Care Med.* 2006;34(8):2113-2119.

[71] Gill PS, Kamath A, Gill TS. Distraction: an assessment of smartphone usage in health care work settings. *Risk Manag. Healthc Policy* 2012;5:105-114.

[72] Shojania KG, Jennings A, Mayhew A, et al. The effects of on-screen, point of care computer reminders on processes and outcomes of care. *Cochrane Database Syst. Rev.* 2009(3):CD001096.

[73] Herasevich V, Kor DJ, Li M, et al. ICU data mart: a non-iT approach. A team of clinicians, researchers and informatics personnel at the Mayo Clinic have taken a homegrown approach to building an ICU data mart. *Healthc Inform* 2011;28(11):42, 44-45.

[74] Herasevich V, Ellsworth MA, Hebl JR, et al. Information Needs for the OR and PACU Electronic Medical Record. *Applied Clinical Informatics* 2014;5(3):630-641.

[75] Brewer T, Colditz GA. Postmarketing surveillance and adverse drug reactions: current perspectives and future needs. *JAMA* 1999;281(9):824-829.

[76] Resar R, Pronovost P, Haraden C, et al. Using a bundle approach to improve ventilator care processes and reduce ventilator-associated pneumonia. *Jt Comm J. Qual Patient Saf* 2005;31(5):243-248.

[77] Sackett DL, Rosenberg WM, Gray JA, et al. Evidence based medicine: what it is and what it isn't. *Bmj* 1996;312(7023):71-72.

[78] Sackett DL. Evidence-based medicine: Wiley Online Library; 2000.

[79] Blumenthal D, Tavenner M. The "meaningful use" regulation for electronic health records. *N. Engl. J. Med.* 2010;363(6):501-504.

[80] Mamlin BW, Biondich PG, Wolfe BA, et al. Cooking up an open source EMR for developing countries: OpenMRS - a recipe for successful

collaboration. AMIA Annual Symposium proceedings / AMIA Symposium *AMIA Symposium* 2006:529-533.

[81] Pickering BW, Herasevich V, Ahmed A, et al. Novel Representation of Clinical Information in the ICU – Developing User Interfaces which Reduce Information Overload. *Applied Clinical Informatics* 2010;1(2):116-131.

[82] Ahmed A, Chandra S, Herasevich V, et al. The effect of two different electronic health record user interfaces on intensive care provider task load, errors of cognition, and performance. *Crit. Care Med.* 2011;39(7):1626-1634.

[83] Yealy DM, Kellum JA, Huang DT, et al. A Randomized Trial of Protocol-Based Care for Early Septic Shock. *New England Journal of Medicine* 2014; 370(18):1683-1693.

[84] Goal-Directed Resuscitation for Patients with Early Septic Shock. *N. Engl. J. Med.* 2014.

[85] Calkin S. Call for a greater focus on sepsis. *Nurs Times* 2014;110(37):2-3.

[86] Abdellatif A, Gunther C, Peppler C, et al. A rare case of splenic abscess with septic peritonitis in a German shepherd dog. *BMC Vet. Res.* 2014;10(1):201.

[87] Bellissimo-Rodrigues WT, Menegueti MG, Gaspar GG, et al. Effectiveness of a Dental Care Intervention in the Prevention of Lower Respiratory Tract Nosocomial Infections among Intensive Care Patients: A Randomized Clinical Trial. *Infect Control Hosp Epidemiol* 2014;35(11):1342-1348.

[88] Herasevich V, Kor DJ, Subramanian A, et al. Connecting the dots: rule-based decision support systems in the modern EMR era. *J. Clin. Monit. Comput* 2013.

[89] AHRQ. *Failure to rescue*. PSNET 2014.

[90] Silber JH, Williams SV, Krakauer H, et al. Hospital and patient characteristics associated with death after surgery. A study of adverse occurrence and failure to rescue. *Med. Care* 1992;30(7):615-629.

[91] Silber JH, Rosenbaum PR, Schwartz JS, et al. Evaluation of the complication rate as a measure of quality of care in coronary artery bypass graft surgery. *JAMA* 1995;274(4):317-323.

[92] Silber JH, Kennedy SK, Even-Shoshan O, et al. Anesthesiologist board certification and patient outcomes. *Anesthesiology* 2002;96(5):1044-1052.

[93] Aiken LH, Clarke SP, Cheung RB, et al. Educational levels of hospital nurses and surgical patient mortality. *JAMA* 2003;290(12):1617-1623.
[94] Wakeam E, Hevelone ND, Maine R, et al. Failure to rescue in safety-net hospitals: availability of hospital resources and differences in performance. *JAMA Surg.* 2014;149(3):229-235.
[95] Silber JH, Rosenbaum PR, Ross RN, et al. Template Matching for Auditing Hospital Cost and Quality. *Health Serv Res* 2014.
[96] Schramm GE, Kashyap R, Mullon JJ, et al. Septic shock: a multidisciplinary response team and weekly feedback to clinicians improve the process of care and mortality. *Crit. Care Med.* 2011;39(2):252-258.
[97] Gaudard M, Ramsey P, Stephens M. Interactive data mining and design of experiments: the JMP® partition and custom design platforms. *North Haven Group* 2006.
[98] Nachimuthu SK, Haug PJ. Early Detection of Sepsis in the Emergency Department using Dynamic Bayesian Networks. *AMIA Annual Symposium proceedings / AMIA Symposium AMIA Symposium* 2012;2012:653-662.
[99] Gultepe E, Green JP, Nguyen H, et al. From vital signs to clinical outcomes for patients with sepsis: a machine learning basis for a clinical decision support system. *Journal of the American Medical Informatics Association : JAMIA* 2013.
[100] Zhou S-M, Gan JQ. Low-level interpretability and high-level interpretability: a unified view of data-driven interpretable fuzzy system modelling. *Fuzzy Sets and Systems* 2008;159(23):3091-3131.

In: Septic Shock
Editor: Benedict Graver

ISBN: 978-1-63463-916-3

Chapter II

Severe Sepsis and Septic Shock: Different Concepts of Analgesia and Sedation May Have Important Influences on Prognosis and Therapy Management

Sven Suefke, Hasib Djonlagić and Thomas Kibbel*
Medical Department I, University Clinic
Schleswig-Holstein, Luebeck, Germany

Introduction

Background: In the scope of analgesia and sedation in intensive care medicine fentanyl was more and more replaced by sufentanil in Europe. Conversely, fentanyl is still more usual worldwide. Furthermore, several advances in the therapy of sepsis were reported. For example, the short-acting

* Corresponding author: Thomas Kibbel, Medical Department I, University Clinic Schleswig-Holstein, Campus Luebeck, Ratzeburger Allee 160, D-23538 Luebeck, Germany. E-mail: th.kibbel@gmx.de.

ß-blocker esmolol showed positive effects in septic shock. However, for analgesia and sedation in this study a combination of sufentanil and propofol was used. Therefore the question arises whether different results can be expected already because of respectively given analgesics or sedatives.

Methods: Because the change has been completed in our institution we examined the data of our transition period from fentanyl/midazolam (F/M) to sufentanil/midazolam (S/M) retrospectively. As such, 2x12 comparable patients (2x 7 males/5 females, age 50-85 years, 2x3 severe sepsis und 2x9 septic shock) had received either only F/M or only S/M for analgesia and sedation. All accordingly to relevant parameters blind recruited patients were analyzed. The therapeutic aim was (1) the best possible tolerance of intensive care by (2) acceptable compatibility of the used drugs.

On the ground of comparable sedation blood pressure, heart rate, laboratory parameters, figures of blood gas analysis and figures of heart rate variability (HRV) were comparatively examined (F/M vs. S/M). For measuring we chose the hour of minimal HRV. At this time the CRP as well as the dose of analgesia and sedation was the highest. Furthermore, an explorative correlation analysis was performed.

Results: Accordingly to the defined therapy target higher analgesic equivalent doses could be given when sufentanil was used ($p<0.001$). Simultaneously, lower midazolam doses had become necessary because of sedative properties of sufentanil by itself ($p=0.008$). Oxygenation could be better performed under S/M (pO_2: $p<0.001$; SO_2: $p=0.005$). Mean blood pressure was less depressed under S/M ($p=0.006$), and the central venous pressure as well ($p=0.015$). On the other hand, heart rate was less elevated under F/M ($p=0.046$). In HRV analysis higher figures of VLF power were found when S/M was used (ln: $p=0.006$). The LF/HF ratio showed vagal predominance in both regimes. However, this was more expressed when F/M was given (0.15 vs. 0.25, $p=0.014$). Further higher values in S/M use were: serum glucose ($p=0.01$), insulin application ($p=0.002$), and body temperature ($p=0.015$). Mortality under infusion or during overhang amounts to 50% in F/M and to 8 % in S/M ($p=0.025$).

Correlation analysis: A clear inverse connection between heart rate and HRV was found overall: vagal determined parameters ($p\leq0.001$) more than global parameters ($p<0.03$). By contrast, only in F/M use (not in S/M use) we found significant associations between metabolic values in the sense of an energetically inefficient anaerobic metabolism: serum glucose vs. serum lactate ($r_P=0.745$; $p=0.005$) and pCO_2 vs. pO_2/serum glucose ($r_S=0.713$; $p=0.009$). Remarkably, similar coherences that can rather be interpreted as centrally induced dynamic adaptations were only seen when S was used (and not when F/M was used): serum glucose vs. LF/HF ratio (r_P=0.758; p=0.004), systolic blood pressure vs. lnVLF (r_P=0.736; p=0.006), pO_2/FiO_2 vs. lnVLF (r_P=0.705; p=0.01), body temperature vs. SDNN (r_P=–0.703; p=0.011) and SO_2 vs. lnTotal Power (r_P=0.666; p=0.018).

Conclusion: The figures from corrclation analysis gave hints that the central autonomic regulation will be better preserved by sufentanil/midazolam than by fentanyl/midazolam. The different mortality can be thoroughly explained by the found discrepancies in that period of time when a direct opioid influence is to suppose. As such, the investigation shows that different concepts of analgesia and sedation may have important influences on risk estimating, on therapy management and on prognosis overall. Statements without specification should be re-questioned.

Background

Whereas fentanyl in the frame of analgesia and sedation in intensive care was widely replaced by sufentanil in central Europe [1, 2], this is not so worldwide. As such, sufentanil plays now as before at most only a subordinate part looking upon the newest US guidelines [3].

In Northern America always mainly morphine, hydromorphone, methadone and fentanyl are commonly used as analgesics. By contrast, e.g., hydromorphone will be not used anymore in Germany and sufentanil was at no time easily available in the United Kingdom.

Besides of such differences in analgesia and sedation, diverse interesting studies exist accordingly to patients with sepsis that have shown on the one hand, that autonomic functions will be typically impaired by severe sepsis and septic shock [4, 5]. This can be ascertained, for example, by decrease of heart rate variability (HRV) [4, 6]. And hereby in one study not the LF/HF ratio in HRV analysis had greatest prognostic relevance as should perhaps rather expected [7, 8],]; surprisingly this was the VLF compartment in frequency domain [9]. And on the other hand in a further relevant study was recently published that frequency control by the short acting ß-blocker esmolol may have positive effects in patients with severe sepsis and septic shock [10]. However, it must not be overlooked that in the two relevant studies was used for analgesia either exclusively fentanyl [9] or exclusively sufentanil [10].

This is only mentioned in the respective methodical parts. Possible consequences even upon the used opioid were not discussed in both works.

Therefore the question is open, whether differences in outcome may be expected already because of different analgesics. Unfortunately, the clearance of this concern has been accompanied by the difficulty that the exchange from fentanyl to sufentanil can regarded as has been finished in central Europe [1, 2].

Table 1. Theoretical advantages of sufentanil in comparison to fentanyl

5-10 fold greater analgesia
greater sedative-hypnotic effect
less cumulation and better steering ability
100 fold greater therapeutic breadth
less respiratory depression
greater hemodynamic stability
less organ toxicity
shorter weaning phase

This replacement was justified by the commonly favorable profile of effects and adverse effects of sufentanil in comparison to fentanyl (Table 1) [11-14]. However, it was always neglected to illustrate the theoretical advantages in practical therapeutic concern.

Additionally, e.g., guidelines on analgesia and sedation in Germany have become much differentiated and as such very complex in the last years [2, 15]. Stiff pattern are here not admissible any longer. Therefore, controlled prospective studies in the concern of the above signified question may be hardly conducted in Europe now. On the other hand on the American continent there was also not seen the urgency on clearing what concept is the best for the patient. In strict contemplation, the recent US guidelines are furthermore basing on the evaluation of the procedures that are performed in practice [3]. Therefore, considerations on principle that are exceeding the frame of the usually done treatment of course cannot be included. Nevertheless, the pharmacological effects of such agents on physiological functions are enormously important.

As such, mortality was higher in elderly patients with arthrosis and rheumatoid arthritis when were treated with opioids [16]. Furthermore can be pointed to the actual problems by hydromorphone/midazolam without sepsis and without respiration [17]. The executed person died after 24 min by retarded and not satisfied demand of oxygen. And questionable effects responsible for should not be referred to midazolam that was given only in a dose that was twice of receiving in colonoscopy; influences of the opioid are more likely.

In the presence of all the above mentioned difficulties, yet we searched for a way for improving the data situation in this concern.

As such we evaluated two data sets from the years 1996-1998 retrospectively. The conception was prospective, but the publication was not performed until now because of capacity limitation. In that time fentanyl as such as sufentanil was - and so is until today on principle – allowed to be used in Germany [1, 2]. However, more fortunately was for that period that on the ground of the formerly guidelines rather comparative collectives could be formed. As such, all patients were usually either ventilated by biphasic positive-airway-pressure (BIPAP) or by synchronized-intermittent-mandatory-ventilation (SIMV) mode for ≥48 hs using the ventilator system Evita® 4 edition, Dräger AG Lübeck, Germany. Aim of the subsequent described investigation was to find out whether perhaps already different opioids may exert different relevant influences on the therapeutic result.

Methods

A) Fundamentals of the Study

For making the comparison possible all patients were treated on customary guidelines. As such, the physiological data were recorded routinely every hour, ca. all 4 hours the values of blood gas analysis were ascertained and two times a day at least the laboratory chemical data. Additionally, a continuous analysis instrument of heart rate variability (HRV) was introduced. The intensity of analgesia conformed to the individual requirement and compatibility in the sense of the Behavioral Pain Scale (BPS), which was developed for uncommunicative patients [18]. Augmentatively, the sedation took place on the Ramsay-Score and the Glasgow-Coma-Scale, respectively.

Aspired was a Ramsay-Score value of 2-3, but this was often exceeded because of already disease connected impairment.

For the period of change (1996-1998) we screened our received data. Because of restriction on the narrow space of time structural falsifications as such as alterations in therapeutic aims should be less probable. Patients were included with severe sepsis and septic shock. Further pre-condition was that for analgesia only fentanyl or only sufentanil was used. Other opioids or the use of both agents led to exclusion. For sedation only midazolam must be given. Other preparations like barbiturates, clonidine or ketamine but also propofol led to exclusion as well. The primary aim of the investigation was to receive the best possible comparison between fentanyl and sufentanil. Because prognosis of sepsis is also dependent on age [19, 20], we restricted our evaluation to patients with an age between 50-85 years.

On the ground of the so given rules we are able to find 2x12 septic patients. Until this stage of investigation it was not even secondary looked on the later evaluated figures. Moreover, all 24 patients that were at first included into the study took part of the calculation. This means that a selection-bias should be also less probable. For the proof of equality we confirmed first the similar starting conditions. This was the basis for any further evaluation.

B) Diagnosis and Therapy

The diagnosis of severe sepsis or septic shock was obtained by clinical and laboratory markers [21]. For evaluation of severity of illness we used the Mortality Probability Model 2nd version at admission (MPM II_0) [22]. The required volume replacement therapy was mainly performed by cristalloide solutions with regard to published recommendations [23]. Catecholamines were applied dependent on the individual state, on the need and on the response of application. In most cases norepinephrine was preferred; this is in accordance with general orders [21].

Likewise, antimicrobial therapy was conducted in adequate dosage [24] and, furthermore, by monitoring the C-reactive protein (CRP) [25, 26]. As antibiotic agents mainly cephalosporines (ceftriaxone, ceftazidime), fluoroquinolones (ciprofloxacin, levofloxacin), macrolides (erythromycin, clarithromycin), imipenem/cilastatin, vancomycin, gentamycin, and metronidazole were used and as antimycotic agent fluconazole. In the case if the initial conducted therapy could not be supposed to be ultimately effective (re-increase of the CRP), the antibiotic regime was changed to other agents.

All patients should be best possible analgesic treated because of disease associated unpleasantness. Analgesia was augmented by sedation on Ramsay-Score. The aim was a value of 2-3 (s. above). Hereby patients should tolerate their functional disorders as well as the therapeutic procedures. Simultaneously, overdoses should be avoided so that the hemodynamic impairment should better controlled by the medical personnel. Overall, in monitoring should be achieved accordantly to the usual guidelines e. g. (1) a central venous pressure (CVP) of 8-12 mmHg, (2) a mean blood pressure of >65 mmHg, (3) a heart rate of 80-90/min as well as (4) a diuresis of >0.5 mL/kg body weight/hour [27, 28].

For this purpose the perfusors of 50 mL were filled with 0.5 mg F, 0.75 mg S or 200 mg M. The then applied dosages oriented first to our own experience data or to instructions from the literature; however, these are not always consistent. For example, 30-100 μg/h in F [29], 10-50 μg/h in S [40], and 10-20 mg/h in midazolam [30] are recommended when patients with normal body weight are concerned (ca. 70 kg). Boluses were not given because patients got mostly to be intubated and therefore treated with a combination of etomidate, fentanyl and midazolam. Basically, analgesia/sedation began with low dosages of opioids and midazolam that were elevated continuously (= titrated) to the desired level [31, 32]. This retarded proceeding was performed to minimize the risk of blood pressure decrease and bradycardia that may occur by too rapid infusions [33, 34], and for reducing the respiratory depressant effects caused by increased thorax rigidity as well [35, 36].

C) Monitoring Procedures

As already mentioned above, continuous monitoring was conducted during the whole course of therapy. Herein the online recording of physiological parameters as well as the intermittent measurement of customary laboratory parameters was conducted. Furthermore, blood gas analysis was done on rather individual requirement (initially about all 4 hours) by using the analyzer system AVL Omni® 9, Roche Diagnostics, Graz, and innovatively the HRV was online recorded ("Cardiovision" multitechmed (MTM) Huenfelden, Germany). The print of the HRV state in time and frequency domain was performed by hourly means. On that basis sympathetic and vagal parts of function and dysfunction, respectively, can be differentiated.

D) Proceeding of the Study

The evaluation of relevant data was done by the following scheme:

1 At first we looked for the period of treatment when dosage of analgesia and sedation was maximal. The CRP was maximal in that space of time too.
2 In the intention of further specification the hour was ascertained in that the HRV showed the lowest values. One can assume that the acute risks for the patient were here greatest at that time.
3 So the time was defined in that all parameters should be contrary evaluated. Until now no concrete insight to the data happened.
4 The substance related comparison of all blind recruited monitoring figures was performed next. This also held true for potential co-factors.
5 In the last step we researched exploratory whether and which agent specific coherences could be find out between the ascertained parameters.

In the concern of the at last conducted correlation analysis we imagined that infectious influences in both use groups were comparable (similar case-mix in subsequently following time periods). This was so also confirmed. Furthermore, the therapy aims as such as the setting like staff, instruments and remedies were widely the same. As such, discrepancies should not only be seen directly upon measured parameters but also upon different connections between the respective parameters, if such should be really relevant in the use of fentanyl or sufentanil.

E) Statistical Analysis

All continuous data that were analyzed by IBM®SPSS® statistics version 21.0 (Somers NY; US) are expressed as mean ± standard deviation. Categorical data given in frequencies were compared with the χ^2-test. The Kolmogorov-Smirnov-test was performed for detection whether the figures are normally distributed or not.

The comparison of parameters between the groups was performed by using the student-t-test for parametric conditions and by using the Mann-Whiteney-U-test for nonparametric conditions.

Because of skewed distribution in HRV parameters a natural logarithmic transformation was performed in frequency domain (except LF/HF) before statistical analysis. The association between the parameters was carried out by Pearson´s correlation (r_P) or by Spearman´s correlation (r_S), respectively. A p-value <0.05 was considered to be statistically significant.

Results

A) Proof of Equivalence in Basic Data and Comparable Results

Table 1 demonstrates that both groups (F and S analgesia) were really comparable from the basic data. The similar held true for the examined depth of sedation according to the Ramsay-Sedation-Scale (3.9 ± 1 vs. 3.8 ± 0.7). Also some parameters on ventilation did not show relevant differences. Similar held true for serum lactate although the values rather tended to be higher when sufentanil was used. And accordingly to catecholamine application no difference could be ascertained between the groups. Also the incidence of arrhythmias gave no hints that would have led to relevant differences in outcome (overall $p<0.1$).

B) Differences between Fentanyl/Midazolam and Sufentanil/ Midazolam

Whereas in first view no substantial differences seemed to exist (Table 2), however, in second view there are indeed remarkable differences between the fentanyl group and the sufentanil group (Table 3). As such, for example, it was possible to give higher analgesic equivalent doses when using sufentanil ($p<0.001$). Simultaneously, lower sedative doses of midazolam were necessary for achieving the same grade of sedation ($p=0.008$ after adjustment to body weight).

Table 2. Basic data and results without significant differences

		Fentanyl	Sufentanil	p
Basic data				
N		12	12	
Male/female		7/5	7/5	
Age [years]		69.7 ± 11.6	68.8 ± 9	n. s.
Body weight [kg]		74.8 ± 11.6	76.9 ± 10.1	n. s.
MPM II_0 [%]		64.4 ± 14.9	63.8 ± 18.3	n. s.
SIRS criteria		3.5 ± 0.7	3.7 ± 0.5	n. s.
CRP maximum [mmol/L]		226 ± 95	234 ± 99	n. s.
Severe sepsis (≥ 1 organ failure)		25 %	25 %	n. s.
Septic shock		75 %	75 %	
Antibiotic and fungizide therapy				
β-Lactam antibiotics		7	10	n. s.
Fluoroquinolones		5	3	
Macrolides		4	4	
Aminoglycosides		4	2	
Vancomycin		6	9	
Fluconazole		7	6	
Depth of sedation				
Ramsay-Sedation-Scale		3.9 ± 1	3.8 ± 0.7	n. s.
Ventilation				
Mode of ventilation	BIPAP	58 %	67 %	n. s.
	SIMV	42 %	33 %	
Ventilation frequency [/min]		11.6 ± 2.2	11.2 ± 2	n. s.
FiO_2 [%]		42.9 ± 13.7	41.3 ± 12.3	n. s.
pCO_2 [mmHg] arterial		41.6 ±8.8	42.7 ± 6.8	n. s.
pH arterial		7.33 ± 0.08	7.33 ± 0.06	n. s.
Lactate generation				
Serum lactate [mmol/L]		3.7 ± 3.5	4.4 ± 2.9	n. s.
Circulation support				
Volume substitution [mL/h]		104 ± 43	101 ± 34	n. s.
Dopamine and/or dobutamine		33 %	33 %	n. s.
Norepinephrine and/or epinephrine < 2mg/h		33 %	42 %	
Norepinephrine and/or epinephrine ≥ 2mg/h		33 %	25 %	
Energy supply				
Glucose 50% p. inf. [mL/h]		26 ± 6	24 ± 5	n. s.
Arrhythmia incidence				
Supraventricular extrasystoles (SVEs), maximum in 24 hs		1492 ± 1384	1024 ± 1513	n. s.
Ventricular extrasystoles (VEs), maximum in 24 hs		279 ± 353	240 ± 305	n. s.
Heart rate variability				
Total Power (TP) [/sec^2]		10.9 ± 9.8	15.2 ± 13.5	>0.1 (ln)
LF [/sec^2]		0.9 ± 1.3	1.5 ± 2.4	>0.1 (ln)
HF [/sec^2]		6.8 ± 6.1	6.4 ± 9.2	>0.5 (ln)
SDNN [/sec]		7.2 ± 2.4	8.6 ± 2.7	>0.1
rMSSD [/sec]		8.3 ± 2.6	7.9 ± 2.2	>0.5
Outcome				
In-hospital mortality		9 (75 %)	5 (42 %)	0.1

Table 3. Results with significant differences

	Fentanyl	Sufentanil	p
Doses of analgesia/sedation			
Maximal F or S dosage [µg/kg/h]	0.723 ± 0.307	0.496 ± 0.263	0.065
Analgesia equivalence (S > 5 x F)		> 2.479 ± 1315	<0.001
Midazolam [mg/kg/h]	0.428 ± 0.158	0.261 ± 0.12	0.008
Oxygenation			
pO_2 [mmHg] arterial	75 ± 11.8	111.7±28.8	<0.001
SO_2 arterial [%]	94.3 ± 1.6	96.5 ± 1.9	0.005
pO_2/ventilation frequency	6.7 ± 2	10.3 ± 3.3	0.005
pO_2/FiO_2 (Horowitz quotient/100)	2 ± 0.9	3 ± 1.1	0.023
pO_2/ventilation frequency x pO_2/FiO_2	14.4 ± 11.7	32.3 ± 20.4	0.015
Blood pressure			
Systolic blood pressure [mmHg]	101 ± 9	112 ± 10	0.012
Diastolic blood pressure [mmHg]	46 ± 6	54 ± 9	0.019
Mean blood pressure [mmHg]	64 ± 6	74 ± 9	0.006
Central venous pressure (CVP) [mmHg]	6.8 ± 1.6	8.6 ± 1.6	0.015
Heart rate and heart rate variability			
Heart rate [/min]	93 ± 21	109 ± 18	0.046
VLF [/sec^2]	1.6 ± 1.4	5.7 ± 5	0.006 (ln)
LF/HF	0.15 ± 0.07	0.25 ± 0.12	0.014
Body temperature [°C]	36.9 ± 0.6	37.7 ± 0.9	0.015
Glucose metabolism			
Serum glucose [mg/dL]	206 ± 53	291 ± 89	0.01
Insulin application [IU/kg/h]	0.028 ± 0.025	0.064 ± 0.026	0.002
Outcome			
Mortality under or ≤ 2 days after infusion	6 (50 %)	1 (8 %)	0.025

Furthermore must be notified that oxygenation could be better performed by sufentanil; oxygen partial pressure (pO_2) and oxygen saturation (SO_2) showed figures that should be advantageous for sufentanil ($p<0.001$ and $p=0.005$, respectively). Similar held true when figures were adjusted to respiratory frequency or to inspiratory oxygen concentration.

Likewise, the blood pressure was not so negative influenced by sufentanil (mean blood pressure: $p=0.006$; central venous pressure: $p=0.015$). Accordingly to heart rate and its variability could be found that heart rate was minor increased by fentanil ($p=0.046$). Figures upon HRV were low in both groups; however, in comparison the VLF compartment and the LF/HF ratio was lower when fentanyl was given ($p=0.006$ and $p=0.014$, respectively).

The body temperature was higher in the sufentanil group ($p=0.015$); also the glucose concentration in serum was higher in the sufentanil group ($p=0.01$) by, moreover remarkably, higher doses of insulin ($p=0.002$).

Parallel to these findings on the ground of only 2x12 septic patients the mortality was higher in the fentanyl group under direct influence of the opioid (i.e., in application phase and in overhang: p=0.025).

According to the causes leading to death in the respective certificates of death was ascertained that under analgesic/sedative agents in each opioid group 1 patient died by respiratory failure. The further 5 under fentanyl were 1 asystole by complete AV block, 3 bradycardic or arhythmogenic circulation failure and 1 cardio-respiratory insufficiency.

C) Correlations in Fentanyl/Midazolam vs. Correlations in Sufentanil/Midazolam

As is already known, the heart rate at rest is more vagal than sympathetic determined [37, 38]. Accordingly, heart rate correlated with HRV inversely in both substances and those interferences were more expressed in vagal activity representing parameters (for example see Figure 1) than in global parameters (Table 4).

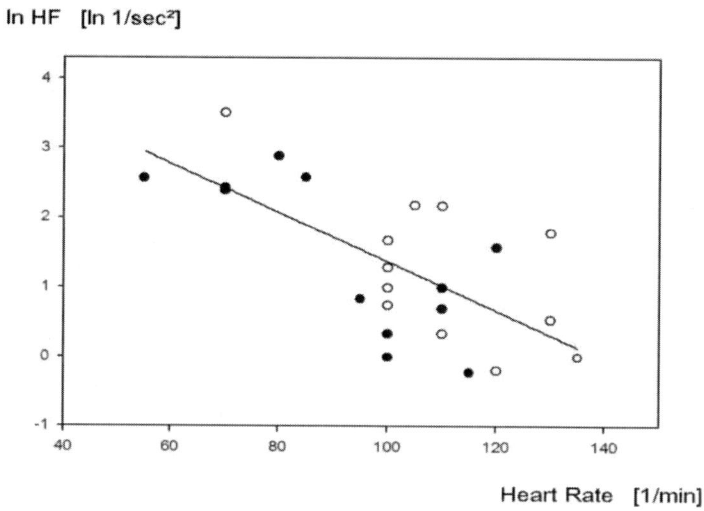

Figure 1. Pearson correlation (r_P) of heart rate with ln HF (fentanyl black, sufentanil white).

Table 4. Pearson Correlation (r_p) of heart rate

	Fentanyl	p	Sufentanil	p	all	p
Total Power (ln)	-0.694	0.012	-0.631	0.028	-0.458	0.024
SDNN	-0.658	0.02	-0.709	0.01	-0.517	0.01
HF (ln)	-0.746	0.005	-0.751	0.005	-0.675	<0.001
rMSSD	-0.694	0.012	-0.749	0.005	-0.655	0.001

However, the correlation coefficients (r_P) were lower overall than that of both single uses. By contrast, the p-values were on the level of single use surely because of greater patient size.

In contrast to heart rate, other connections were not the same in the fentanyl group and the sufentanil group if they were found at all.

At first, our interests pointed to the VLF component of power because this parameter exerted the greatest predictive value in sepsis when fentanyl for analgesia and midazolam or propofol for sedation was used [9]. Surprisingly, we found here clear associations with further monitoring parameters when sufentanil was used (Table 5) but not when fentanyl was used.

Similar, for example, held also true for the LF/HF ratio that has proved in other studies to be important in ICU patients [7, 8, 39]. The association of LF/HF with serum glucose (Figure 2) was also found in the respective glucose level variation (see below).

The second best correlation was found between the VLF component and the systolic blood pressure (Figure 3).

Table 5. Pearson Correlations (r_p) of HRV paramerters with physiological parameters

HRV parameter	Correlated parameter	Fentanyl	p	Sufentanil	p
LF/HF ratio	Serum glucose	-0.112	n.s.	+0.758	0.004
ln VLF	Systolic blood pressure	-0.211	n.s.	+0.736	0.006
ln VLF	pO_2/FiO_2	0.092	n.s.	0.705	0.01
SDNN	Body temperature	+0.545	0.067	-0.703	0.011
ln Total Power	SO_2 arterial	0.067	n.s.	0.666	0.018
ln VLF	SO_2 arterial	0.354	n.s.	0.626	0.03
LF/HF ratio	pO_2/ventilation frequency	0.131	n.s.	0.597	0.04

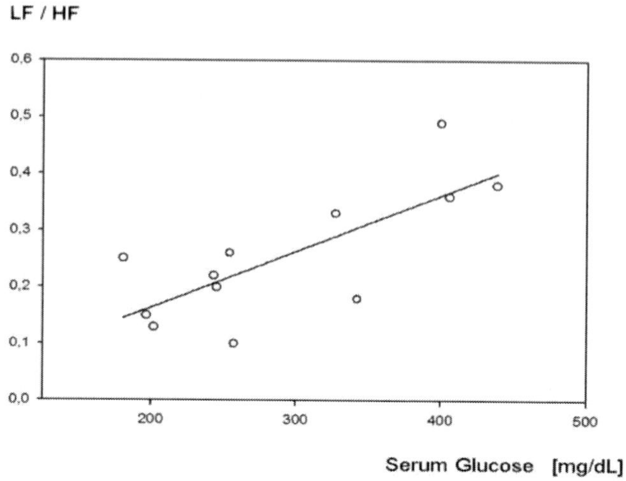

Figure 2. Pearson correlation (r_P) of LF/HF ratio and serum glucose in sufentanil/ midazolam use.

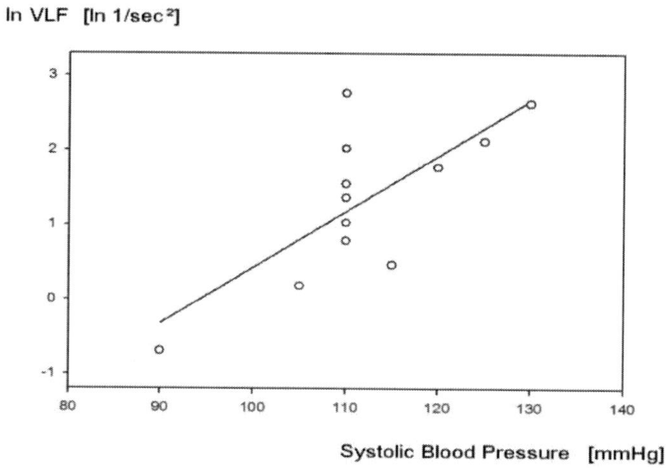

Figure 3. Pearson correlation (r_P) of ln VLF and systolic blood pressure in sufentanil/ midazolam use.

Remarkably, such coherences could not be seen when fentanyl/midazolam was used. In contrast to sufentanil, another pattern was present when fentanyl was given. Here existed clear connections between such parameters that are in accordance with an anaerobic metabolism. As such, lactate correlated with serum glucose (Table 6 and Figures 4/5).

Table 6. Pearson/Spearman Correlations (r_P, r_S) with regard to anaerobic metabolism

Correlated parameters		Fentanyl	p	Sufentanil	p
Serum glucose	Lactate	0.745 (r_P)	0.005	0.444 (r_P)	n.s.
pH	Lactate	-0.163 (r_P)	n.s.	-0.767 (r_P)	0.004
pO_2	pCO_2	0.615 (r_S)	0.033	-0.293 (r_S)	n.s.
Serum glucose	pCO_2	-0.559 (r_S)	0.059	-0.375 (r_S)	n.s.
pO_2/serum glucose	pCO_2	0.713 (r_S)	0.009	0.007 (r_S)	n.s.

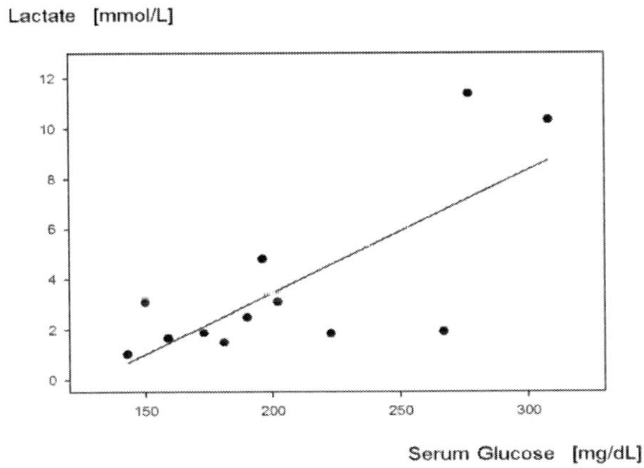

Figure 4. Pearson correlation (r_P) of serum glucose and lactate in fentanyl/midazolam use.

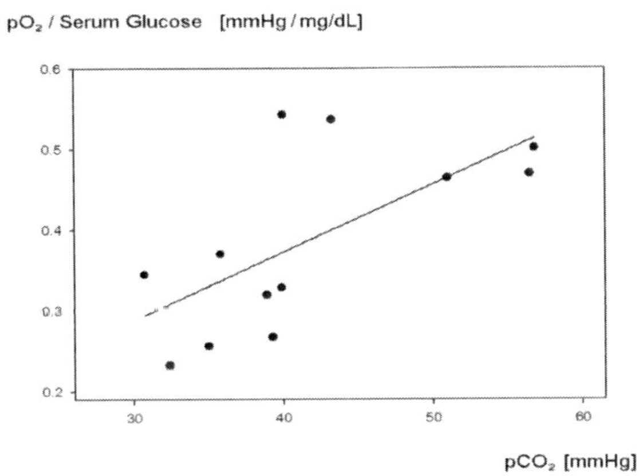

Figure 5. Spearman correlation (r_S) of pO_2/serum glucose and pCO_2 in fentanyl/ midazolam use.

Remarkably, a clear and rather expected connection between lactate and blood pH was seen in the sufentanil group instead of (Figure 6).

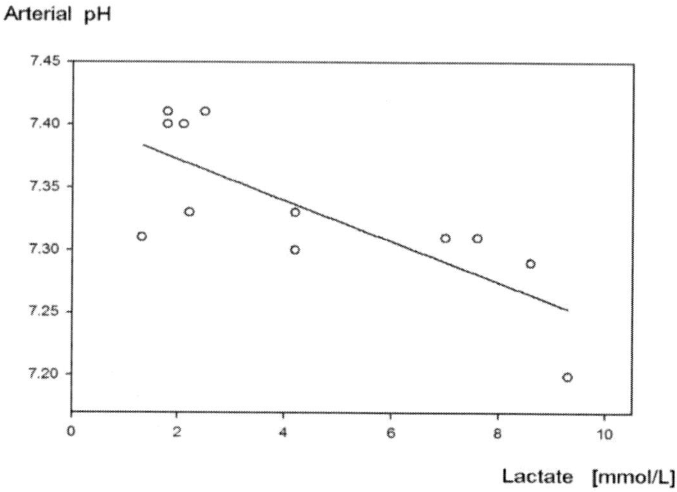

Figure 6. Pearson correlation (r_P) of pH and lactate in sufentanil/midazolam use.

Discussion

A) General Aspects

The regimes for analgesia and sedation are quite different in respiration needing ICU patients worldwide. As such, the respective results on this topic cannot commonly transfered into each other. About this is consensus for more than 10 years [40, 41]. However, basically comparative investigations on the question do not exist what drugs are rather advantageous. And in the high-developed countries of Europe and Northern America every side is developing the respective procedures for its own.

Nevertheless, for getting more knowledge in this concern we investigated our data from that time in that fentanyl and sufentanil were commonly parallel used in Germany and we decided to introduce sufentanil by leaving fentanyl.

Accordingly to sedation we restricted our study on midazolam. Thus, mixed results should be minimal. Moreover, it is not really reasonable, for example, to compare respiration needing strokes after hypertensive crises with septic shocks under catecholamines. As such, we further restricted on latter patients, also because widely homogeneous patient groups with adequate numbers could be recruited. Conversely, this means furthermore that the received results on septic patients cannot be simply transfered to other patient groups.

B) Special Differences between Fentanyl and Sufentanil

The results of our investigation on patients in the age of 55-85 years with severe sepsis or septic shock show in main:

1. Higher analgesic equivalent doses were possible with sufentanil ($p<0.001$; Table 2). Comparatively analgesic doses by fentanyl should probably not have been well tolerated by the treated patients. This aspect is much relevant because a lot of patients have reported that they suffered pain during the treatment. In that, physicians as well as nurses are typically estimating the need of analgesics as too low [42, 43]. By contrast, approximately 75% of ICU patients reported severe pain during their treatment despite more than 80% of the caregivers considered the analgesia to be adequate [44]. However, an adequate monitoring of analgesia is relevant for outcome of critically ill patients that are widely unable to communicate [45].
2. Lower midazolam doses after adjustment to body weight had become necessary by the use of sufentanil for getting the same sedation state on Ramsay score ($p=0.008$; Table 3). This result can be explained by the greater sedative potency of sufentanil by itself [46, 47]. Nevertheless, although midazolam is characterized by a high therapeutic index in general [48, 49], the potential influence of midazolam on respiration and oxygen supply [47, 49] could be minimized when using sufentanil. Similar could be also relevant in view of an imaginable net sympatheticolysis [51, 52].
3. The oxygenation of the blood could be better performed under sufentanil/midazolam than under fentanyl/midazolam in the concept of a greater fentanyl induced thorax rigidity (pO_2: $p<0.001$) [12, 13, 36]. Even after correction upon the ventilation frequency and/or upon the concentration of the inhaled oxygen the difference in pO_2 reached level of significance ($p<0.025$). Similarly, this held true for the arterial SO_2 ($p=0.005$). Such is important for prognosis as a progressive O_2 deficiency also limits myocardial contractility [53].

4. Accordingly to the decrease in blood pressure and heart rate when opioids were given to rabbits in anesthetic doses [54], we found differentially a more reduced blood pressure under fentanyl/midazolam than under sufentanil/midazolam (p=0.006). In such concern was shown that the cardiac output decreased only slightly but significantly under sufentanil in the dog [55]. However, in other trials a negative inotropic effect was found in fentanyl [56] and not so in sufentanil [57].
5. Simultaneously, the heart rate was less elevated under fentanyl/midazolam. Therefore, from the different figures of blood pressure and heart rate can be concluded that not the same size of patients could have been involved in the study of Morelli et al. [10]. In this study was shown that the short acting ß blocker esmolol had positive effects on patients with septic shock when a combination of sufentanil and propofol was used for analgesia/sedation. This regime is quite usual in Italy for a lot of years [1]. However it is not known until now, whether such advantages are independent from the respectively used analgesic agent. Remarkably, in that study only patients were participating that exerted a heart rate of ≥95/min by a simultaneous mean blood pressure of ≥65 mmHg. However, by this inclusion criteria 10 of 12 of our sufentanil patients but only 5 of 12 of our fentanyl patients should have been treated by esmolol (p=0.035). As such, it must be rather expected that already different concepts of analgesia/sedation may have significant influences on therapeutic proceeding and therapeutic results as well. Generalized statements without differentiation on opioids should be re-questioned.
6. The VLF Power component of HRV in one study had greatest prognostic relevance in multiple organ dysfunction syndrome under fentanyl/midazolam or under fentanyl/propofol [9]. Accordingly, in our investigation even this parameter was found to be significantly higher under sufentanil/midazolam (p=0.006). Although the meaning of HRV in very low frequency power (VLF) is widely unsettled [58], nevertheless, there are hints that the density of this frequency component is not only important for prognosis in patients with sepsis [9, 59] but also in such with congestive heart failure [60] or COPD [61]. Therefore, a coherence of oxygen supply and VLF fluctuations can be thoroughly assumed [62]. Furthermore, much interestingly the VLF power after ln-transformation was one of the strongest predictors of outcome in trauma patients with or without traumatic brain injury [63]. Additionally, sedation (surely analgo-sedation is meant) had clear effects on HRV in this study whereas

ß blockers didn´t have. And this study was conducted in Florida where sufentanil most probably was not used [3, 40].

7. Furthermore and remarkably, the second differentiating marker on mortality in the latter study was also the LF/HF [63]. As such, the LF/HF ratio that was also prognostically relevant in other sepsis studies [7, 8], was higher found in our investigation under sufentanil/midazolam than under fentanyl/midazolam, and this although the CRP was comparable. Accordingly is known that a burden of endotoxines will lead to a reduction of beat-to-beat variability over the total spectrum of HRV [4]. Nevertheless, the LF band was the best predictor for multiple organ failure [6] and the HF band was comparatively even higher when patients died later [64]. Therefore, not only the size of HRV diminution should be relevant in sepsis, but likewise especially the LF/HF ratio <1.
8. Moreover, the body temperature was slightly, but significantly higher found under sufentanil/midazolam (0.8°C; $p=0.015$). A decrease of temperature was also seen by an inadequate tissue oxygenation when F was used in abdominal aortic surgery [65]. This all corresponds to the reported decrease of temperature under continuous F infusion within a space of 20 min (0.7°C) [66]. In that concern, one must not overlook that the oxygen demand will be simultaneously reduced by the diminished heart rate [67, 68]. Furthermore, the O_2 consumption decreases by 10-13% in general, when the temperature decreases by 1°C [69]. Indeed, both would surely have had favorable influences on energy balance, but regarding fentanyl it must be queried that such positive effects are equalizing the negative ones caused by hypoxemia.
9. Further is to mention that serum glucose concentration was higher ascertained in the sufentanil group ($p=0.01$) although higher insulin doses were given ($p=0.002$; Table 3). In that concern, greater studies have shown that even higher blood glucose was a general risk marker in intensive care patients [70-72]. However, the aspect of further perhaps more relevant parameters was not considered. Accordingly, energy generation increases to cope with greater metabolic demands that are needed to deal with the acute inflammatory insult [73]. However, when additional impairment of pulmonary function becomes present, no sufficient compensation of oxygenation and tissue perfusion will be reached usually even if respiration is mechanically supported [23]. According to our data it can be surely assumed that the oxygen provision under fentanyl was not optimal. In such preconditions glucose should be more anaerobically metabolized so that more lactate should be formed

[65, 74]. Hereby, the lactate concentration should be gained to a maximum and afterwards the lactate itself will be metabolized as substitute [75, 76].

C) Considerations on currently discussed blood glucose variability

Regarding to recently published results, lower heart rate variability correlated with higher blood glucose variability [77, 78] and both with higher mortality [79-81]. As such we looked after the study has properly finished whether the aspect of more or less variation in blood glucose was perhaps relevant for the study result. As such, we calculated first the standard deviation (SD) of 9 values of serum glucose within 8 hs before maximum of analgesia/sedation until 8 hs after maximum of analgesia/sedation for each patient (4 values before, value of analgesia/sedation maximum, 4 values afterwards). Then the valuation was conducted in the manner as was done before.

Table 7. Serum glucose variation in fentanyl/midazolam vs. sufentanil/midazolam

	Fentanyl	Sufentanil	p
Mean of serum glucose within 16 hs [mg/dL]	197 ± 49	247 ± 58	0.031
SD of serum glucose within 16 hs [mg/dL]	47.5 ± 32.2	49.4 ± 22.7	n.s.
SD of serum glucose within 16 hs / serum glucose at maximal analgesia/sedation	22.1 ± 10.6 %	17.4 ± 7.2 %	n.s.
Elevation of serum glucose at maximal analgesia/sedation regarding to the mean of the 1st,2nd,8th and 9th value [mg/dL]	29 ± 62	75 ± 57	0.03
Elevation of serum glucose at maximal analgesia/sedation vs. mean of the 1st,2nd,8th and 9th value	$p > 0.1$	$p = 0.001$	
Pearson Correlation of SD of serum glucose within 16 hs vs. LF/HF at HRV minimum	$r_P = + 0.740$ $p=0.006$	$r_P = - 0.303$ $p >0.1$	

Accordingly to most non-significant differences of HRV parameters in time and frequency domain we also found no relevant differences in the variation of blood glucose concentration (Table 7). In detail was further shown that serum glucose in mean over the 16 hs was lower than at analgesia/sedation maximum. However, this difference was only significant in the sufentanil group ($p=0.001$). Moreover, in correlation analysis only one relevant connection was found between glucose variation and HRV. As such, only a positive association was only ascertained between the 16 hs SD of glucose and the LF/HF ratio in sufentanil use ($r_P = 0.740$; $p = 0.006$). Also this result could be perhaps interpreted as a better adjustment to the need of necessary energy in sepsis [73] by this substance. Such would be in accordance to Table 5 and Figure 2.

Thus, this coherence only found in the sufentanil group is underlining the suggestion of a better preserved central regulation when sufentanil was applicated (below). Furthermore, this would mean that changes on acute pathophysiological or pharmaceutical conditions must be surely differentiated from glucose variability in not otherwise influenced euglycemic range [81].

Beyond glucose variability, as is mentioned above, it was reported repeatedly that hyperglycemia serves as a special risk factor in critically ill patients [70-72]. By contrast, it was also stated that a stress-induced hyperglycemia acted rather protectively in septic shock [82]. In this concern, the data of Table 7 may show that this discrepancy could be thoroughly declared already on the ground of different opioid analgesia.

D) Correlation Analysis with Respect to Central Autonomic Regulation

In the conception that glucose will be more anaerobical metabolized by relative oxygen deficit under fentanyl (stronger glycolysis, less energy supply), the glucose level should be on the one hand increasingly decreased and on the other hand the minor oxygen should be increasingly used for metabolizing the lactate already because of quantity relation. If this is right, glucose and lactate concentrations must correlate with each other in fentanyl. Even this was confirmed by our data (Figure 4: $r_P = 0.745$; $p=0.005$). Moreover, such connection was more expressed below 200 mg/dL than above 200 mg/dL. Already on the ground of such observed straddle it could be expected that a respective coherence should not be found in sufentanil. Instead of the lactate correlated negatively with arterial blood pH (Figure 6: $r_P = -0.767$, $p = 0.004$).

The more restricted metabolism by fentanyl should be further underlined by the relatively weaker but nevertheless significant connections of pCO_2 and

pO_2 as such as of pCO_2 and serum glucose (inversely). And in combination those associations showed additive importance (Figure 5: $r_S = 0.713$; $p = 0.009$). On the other side the differing associations in sufentanil/midazolam use would mean that the oxygen supply is lower depressed in the respective application. And the better oxygen supply in sufentanil use could serve for the condition that the central regulation was here better preserved than in fentanyl use.

The significantly found coherences of physiological parameters with HRV parameters only in the sufentanil group are in accordance with this assumption (Table 5). The appearently better autonomic regulation prosperities in sufentanil may be declared by the better oxygenation. And the better autonomic regulation may be indirectly responsible for the better homeostasis. Both results (better oxygenation and better central adaptations) may also lead to the further assumption that the energy supply could be more adequately performed by the use of sufentanil/midazolam.

E) Lactate As a Central Risk Marker

The lactate concentration in plasma serves as central parameter in the risk estimation of patients in intensive care [29]. As such, the level was indeed similar in fentanyl and sufentanil use. However, in differentiated consideration this similarity should be rather deceptive. Yet the offer of energy is not possible without oxygen and in hypoxemia glycolysis is preferred. Accordingly, at first an elevated lactate concentration should be expected under the precondition of a generally reduced oxygen supply. This would lead to hypoglycemia. However, by stronger reduction of glucose in the substrate on the ground of excessive generation of lactate we should assume that the residually available oxygen will be rather used for metabolizing the lactate than for metabolizing the remaining glucose. This would mean that the marker lactate will be secondly increasingly reduced and may delude a better state in net as must be supposed by the hypoxemic state. In consequence of this relevant further decomposition of lactate this laboratory parameter should be likely of poorer reliability in the use of fentanyl and the figures should not be simply equalized with that of sufentanil.

F) Outcome Relevance

Although the patient number is low, the different rate of non-survival is then in accordance to the found differences between fentanyl and sufentanil when a direct influence must be supposed (p=0.025). In this concern it must not be neglected that especially fentanyl is cumulated in longer-term therapy and an abrupt stopping of infusion is not leading to effect reduction at the same time. Nevertheless, it is not surprising that this difference diminished over time and difference of mortality in the hospital was ultimately not so discrepant (p=0.1). The momentary perhaps fortunate analgesia/sedation should of course not abolish the already occurred multi-organ impairment.

G) Limitations

In the consideration afterwards, the dosage of midazolam in the fentanyl application that has widely abandoned in Germany surely was relatively high in comparison to actual US recommendations [3]. However, there are also reports about nearly high midazolam doses in sepsis [82] and in the translation of "The ICU Book" of Paul L. Marino the German translators remarked that to their opinion the dosage of midazolam should be too low [29]. On this background no dosage of fentanyl, midazolam or propofol was unfortunately given in the study sponsored by the Deutsche Forschungsgemeinschaft (DFG) [9]. Likewise, also in the study on trauma patients [63] or in the recently published study on esmolol in septic shock no dosages on analgesics and sedatives were reported [10], not to speak of the respective antibiotics that should exert also different influences on autonomic nervous function.

The discrepant glucose levels and insulin supplementations would also lead to further open questions. As such, the study gave no finishing answers how the stronger glycolysis under fentanyl or how the higher glucose levels respectively the higher insulin application under sufentanil must be estimated. However, an overall rather unfortunate effect in fentanyl because of decreased oxygen supply should be probable upon our data.

From the view of today it must be surely criticized that no details on now usual scores of pain and agitation were documented. However, different aim criteria or performed procedures are less probable because of time restriction. On the other hand, in the concern of an intended comparison of agents the absolute figures of scores would play rather only a subordinate role. And that the study patients were analgesic and sedative treated on clear regulations is underlined by the result that significant correlations were at least partly found inter-individually.

A further lack by the knowledge of today is likely given by the fact that indeed the catecholamine supplements were recorded but not so the resulting concentrations in the blood. Although the application of catecholamines was comparable nothing is said about the really achieved equivalents. Because no levels of norepinephrine and epinephrine were ascertained, no final statement can be made. However, the knowledge on this point is desirable in the concern of an eventual disadvantageous feedback mechanism [83]. Such should be carried out in further studies.

By the recently published US guidelines on analgesia and sedation in the critically ill is recommended that for sedation rather propofol than midazolam should be used. This is justified by the less expressed delirium under propofol [3]. However, hereby it must be referred on sepsis that propofol was rather associated with further sympathicolysis [84-86]. Therefore, especially in sepsis further investigation is needed; for the LF/HF ratio is already reduced on the ground of low HRV activity [7, 8].

However, pharmacological valuations are aggravated because data on pure physiological conditions are widely missing. Only some results on HRV alteration under hypoxia and exercise in healthy subjects are published [87-89]. As such, it can be only suggested that central regulations are better preserved by sufentanil. Therefore, more interesting would be to know what coherences in the vitally limited field must be considered. However, ethical scruples can quite quick arise in investigations on strongly endangered patients.

Conclusion

In the contrast of correlations that are rather a sign of an anaerobical metabolism, we found in fentanyl nearly no clear connections of physiological data with HRV parameters. This was just the opposite in sufentanil. The exception was only served by heart rate that correlated in both investigated opioids especially with the vagal determined parameters of HRV.

In sufentanil we found widely no connections between rather stiff figures of metabolism, but instead of connections that can be rather interpreted as acute central adaptation processes. The exception here was the common association between lactate and arterial blood pH.

Because of the ascertained differences can be assumed that the impairment of autonomic nervous system in therapy of sepsis is not only due to alteration by sepsis for its own.

At least such deterioration can be strengthened by analgesics. As such, in a former study was found that the VLF component of frequency domain had greatest predictive value when fentanyl was used for analgesia. And even this component of HRV showed in our study more fortunate figures in sufentanil use. Therefore, the results from that former study cannot be extended to conditions where sufentanil is used. This also holds true for the respective risk estimation on blood glucose level.

In wider concern must be concluded that the results on the ground of different practice in analgesia/sedation cannot be transferred simply e.g., from Europe on North America and conversely. For clearance what agent should rather be given, further investigation is necessary.

Accordingly, the still open questions are of minor interest in central Europe because several advantages are assumed for sufentanil. However, because it must be considered that the therapeutic result in severe sepsis and septic shock will be at least not poorer when sufentanil is used, controlled comparison studies fentanyl vs. sufentanil should be rather justifiable when were conducted out of central Europe.

Conflicts of Interest

None declared.

References

[1] Soliman, H. M.; Mélot, C. and Vincent, J. L. (2001) Sedative and analgesic practice in the intensive care unit: the results of a European survey. *Br. J. Anaesth.*, 87, 186-192.

[2] Martin, J.; Heymann, A.; Bäsell, K.; Baron, R.; Biniek, R.; Bürkle, H.; Dall, P.; Dictus, C.; Eggers, V.; Eichler, I.; Engelmann, L.; Garten, L.; Hartl, W.; Haase, U.; Huth, R.; Kessler, P.; Kleinschmidt, S.; Koppert, W.; Kretz, F. J.; Laubenthal, H.; Marggraf, G.; Meiser, A.; Neugebauer, E.; Neuhaus, U.; Putensen, C.; Quintel, M.; Reske, A.; Roth, B.; Scholz, J.; Schröder, S.; Schreiter, D.; Schüttler, J.; Schwarzmann, G.; Stingele,

R.; Tonner, P., and Tränkle, P. (2010) Evidence and Consensus-based German guidelines for the management of analgesia, sedation and delirium in intensive care – short version. *Ger. Med. Sci.*, 8, Doc02.

[3] Barr, J.; Fraser, G. L.; Puntillo, K.; Ely, E. W; Gélinas, C.; Dasta, J. F.; Davidson, J. E.; Devlin, J. W.; Kress, J. P.; Joffe, A. M.; Coursin, D. B.; Herr, D. L.; Tung, A.; Robinson, B. R.; Fontaine, D. K.; Ramsay, M. A.; Riker, R. R.; Sessler, C. N.; Pun, B.; Skrobik, Y., and Jaeschke, R. (2013) Clinical Practice Guidelines for the Management of Pain, Agitation, and Delirium in Adult Patients in the Intensive Care Unit. *Crit. Care Med.*, 41, 263-306.

[4] Godin, P. J.; Fleisher, L. A.; Eidsath, A.; Vandivier, R. W.; Preas, H. L.; Banks, S. M.; Buchman, T. G., and Suffredini, A. F. (1996) Experimental human endoxemia increases cardiac regularity: results from a prospective, randomized, crossover trial. *Crit. Care Med.*, 24, 1117-1124.

[5] Muller-Werdan, U.; Buerke, M.; Ebelt, H.; Heinroth, K. M.; Herklotz, A.; Loppnow, H.; Ruß, M.; Schlegel, F.; Schlitt, A.; Schmidt, H. B.; Söffker, G., and Werdan, K. (2006) Septic cardiomyopathy – A not yet discovered cardiomyopathy? *Exp. Clin. Cardiol.*, 11, 226-236.

[6] Pontet, J.; Contreras, P.; Curbelo, A.; Medina, J.; Noveri, S.; Bentancourt, S., and Migliaro, E. R. (2003) Heart rate variability as early marker of multiple organ dysfunction syndrome in septic patients. *J. Crit. Care*, 18, 156-163.

[7] Korach, M.; Sharshar, T.; Jarrin, I.; Fouillot, J. P.; Raphaël, J. C.; Gajdos, P., and Annane, D. (2001) Cardiac variability in critically ill adults: Influence of sepsis. *Crit. Care Med.*, 29, 1380-1385.

[8] Barnaby, D.; Ferrick, K.; Kaplan, D. T.; Shah, S.; Bijur, P., and Gallagher, E. J. (2002) Heart rate variability in emergency department patients with sepsis. *Acad. Emerg. Med.*, 9, 661-670.

[9] Schmidt, H.; Müller-Werdan, U.; Hoffmann, T.; Francis, D. P.; Piepoli, M. F.; Rauchhaus, M.; Prondzinsky, R.; Loppnow, H.; Buerke, M.; Hoyer, D., and Werdan, K. (2005) Autonomic dysfunction predicts mortality in patients with multiple organ dysfunction syndrome of different age groups. *Crit. Care Med.*, 33, 1994-2002.

[10] Morelli, A.; Ertmer, C.; Westphal, M.; Rehberg, S.; Kampmeier, T.; Ligges, S.; Orecchioni, A.; D'Egidio, A.; D'Ippoliti, F.; Raffone, C.; Venditti, M.; Guarracino, F.; Girardis, M.; Tritapepe, L.; Pietropaoli, P.; Mebazaa, A., and Singer, M. (2013) Effect of heart rate control with

esmolol on hemodynamic and clinical outcomes in patients with septic shock: a randomized clinical trial. *JAMA*, 310, 1683-1691.

[11] Bailey, P. L.; Streisand, J. B.; East, K. A.; East, T. D.; Isern, S.; Hansen, T. W.; Posthuma, E. F.; Rozendaal, F. W.; Pace, N. L., and Stanley, T. H. (1990) Differences in magnitude and duration of opioid-induced respiratory depression and analgesia with fentanyl and sufentanil. *Anesth. Analg.*, 70, 8-15.

[12] Ellmauer, S. (1994) [Sufentanil. An alternative to fentanyl/alfentanil?] *Anaesthesist*, 43, 143-158.

[13] Prause, A.; Wappler, F.; Scholz, J.; Bause, H., and Schulte am Esch, J. (2000) Respiratory depression under long-term sedation with sufentanil. Midazolam and clonidine has no clinical significance. *Intensive Care Med.*, 26, 1454-1461.

[14] Schaffrath, E.; Kuhlen, R. and Tonner, P. H. (2004) [Analgesia and sedation in intensive care medicine.] *Anaesthesist*, 53, 1111-1132.

[15] Braune, S. and Kluge, S. (2012) Aktuelle Sedierungskonzepte in der Intensivmedizin. *Dtsch. Med. Wochenschr.*, 137, 190-193.

[16] Solomon, D. H.; Rassen, J. A.; Glynn, R. J.; Lee, J.; Levin, R., and Schneeweiss, S. (2010) The comparative safety of analgesics in older adults with arthritis. *Arch. Intern. Med.*, 170, 1968-1976.

[17] Dyer, O. (2014) The slow death of lethal injection. *B. M. J.*, 348, g2670.

[18] Payen, J. F.; Bru, O.; Bosson, J. L.; Lagrasta, A.; Novel, E.; Deschaux, I.; Lavagne, P., and Jacquot, C. (2001) Assessing pain in critically ill sedated patients by using a behavioral pain scale. *Crit. Care Med.*, 29, 2258–63.

[19] Martin, G. S.; Mannino, D. M. and Moss, M. (2006) The effect of age on the development and outcome of adult sepsis. *Crit. Care Med.*, 34, 15-21.

[20] Brunner-Ziegler, S.; Heinze, G.; Ryffel, M.; Kompatscher, M.; Slany, J., and Valentin, A. (2007) "Oldest old" patients in intensive care: prognosis and therapeutic activity. *Wien. Klin. Wochenschr.*, 119, 14-19.

[21] Reinhart, K.; Brunkhorst, F. M.; Bone, H. G.; Gerlach, H.; Gründling, M.; Kreymann, G.; Kujath, P.; Marggraf, G.; Mayer, K.; Meier-Hellmann, A.; Peckelsen, C.; Putensen, C.; Stüber, F.; Quintel, M.; Ragaller, M.; Rossaint, R.; Weiler, N.; Welte, T., and Werdan, K. (2006) [Diagnosis and therapy of sepsis. S-2-Guidelines of the German Sepsis Society Inc. (DSG) and the German Interdisciplinary Society for Intensive and Emergency Medicine (DIVI).] *Anaesthesist*, 55 (Suppl. 1), 43-56.

[22] Lemeshow, S.; Teres, D.; Klar, J.; Avrunin, J. S.; Gehlbach, S. H., and Rapoport, J. (1993) Mortality Probability Models (MPM II) based on an international cohort of Intensive Care Unit patients. *JAMA*, 270, 2478-2486.

[23] Brunkhorst, F. M. and Reinhart, K. (2009) [Supportive and adjunctive sepsis therapy.] *Internist*, 50, 817-827.

[24] Bodmann, K. F. (2005) Current guidelines for the treatment of severe pneumonia and sepsis. *Chemotherapy*, 51, 227-233.

[25] Kepa, L. and Oczko-Grzesik, B. (2001) [Usefulness of plasma C-reactive protein (CRP) estimation in patients with bacterial sepsis.] *Przegl. Epidemiol.*, 55 (Suppl. 3), 63-67.

[26] Schmit, X. and Vincent, J. L. (2008) The time course of blood C-reactive protein concentrations in relation to the response to initial antimicrobial therapy in patients with sepsis. *Infection*, 36, 213-219.

[27] Rivers, E.; Nguyen, B.; Havstad, S.; Ressler, J.; Muzzin, A.; Knoblich, B.; Peterson, E., and Tomlanovich, M. (2001) Early goal-directed therapy in the treatment of severe sepsis and septic shock. *N. Engl. J. Med.*, 345, 1368-1377.

[28] Dellinger, R. P.; Levy, M. M.; Carlet, J. M.; Bion, J.; Parker, M. M.; Jaeschke, R.; Reinhart, K.; Angus, D. C.; Brun-Buisson, C.; Beale, R.; Calandra, T.; Dhainaut, J. F.; Gerlach, H.; Harvey, M.; Marini, J. J.; Marshall, J.; Ranieri, M.; Ramsay, G.; Sevransky, J.; Thompson, B. T.; Townsend, S.; Vender, J. S.; Zimmerman, J. L., and Vincent, J. L. (2006) Surviving Sepsis Campain: International guidelines for management of severe sepsis and septic shock 2008. *Crit. Care Med.*, 36, 1394-1396.

[29] Marino, P. L. (ed.) Das ICU Buch – Praktische Intensivmedizin, German revision by Taeger, K.; Bucher, M.; Drescher, J.; Farnhammer, C.; Fehervary, P.; Göbel, F.; Hansen, E.; Jakob, W.; Kerschbaum, G.; Keyl, C.; Koppenberg, J.; Lemberger, P.; Mertz, M.; Nickl, S.; Prasser, C.; Schickendantz, J.; Schneider, A.; Wegenhorst, U.; Wiesenack, C.; Wülfing-Palizsch and Zimmermann, M.; 2nd ed., *Urban and Schwarzenberg*, München Wien 1998.

[30] Pohlman, A. S.; Simpson, K. P. and Hall, J. B. (1994) Continuous intravenous infusions of lorazepam versus midazolam for sedation during mechanical ventilatory support: a prospective, randomized study. *Crit. Care Med.*, 22, 1241-1247.

[31] Schweickert, W. D. and Kress, J. P. (2008) Strategies to optimize analgesia and sedation. *Crit. Care*, 12 (Suppl. 3), S6.

[32] Gommers, D. and Bakker, J. (2008) Medications for analgesia and sedation in the intensive care unit: an overview. *Crit. Care*, 12 (Suppl. 3), S4.

[33] Laubie, M.; Schmitt, H. and Drouillat, M. (1977) Central sites and mechanisms of the hypotensive and bradycardic effects of the narcotic anagesic agent fentanyl. *Naunyn Schmiedebergs Arch. Pharmacol.*, 296, 255-2619.

[34] Levine, R. L. (1994) Pharmacology of intravenous sedatives and opioids in critically ill patients. *Crit. Care Clin.*, 10, 709-731.

[35] Waldvogel, H. H. (ed.) Analgetika, Antinozizeptiva, Adjuvanzien. Teil B: Allgemeine Pharmakologie zentraler Schmerzmittel, Zentrale Analgetika: Opioide. Springer, Berlin Heidelberg New York 1996.

[36] Streisand, J. B.; Bailey, P. L.; LeMaire, L.; Ashburn, M. A.; Tarver, S. D.; Varvel, J., and Stanley, T. H. (1993) Fentanyl-induced rigidity and unconsciousness in human volunteers. Incidence, duration, and plasma concentrations. *Anesthesiology*, 78, 629-634.

[37] Nyberg, G. (1981) Vagal and sympathetic contributions to the heart rate at rest and during isometric and dynamic exercise in young healthy men. *J. Cardiovasc. Pharmacol.*, 3, 1243-50.

[38] Langewitz, W.; Rüddel, H.; Schächinger, H.; Lepper, W.; Mulder, L. J.; Veldman, J. H., and van Roon, A. (1991) Changes in sympathetic and parasympathetic cardiac activation during mental load: an assessment by spectral analysis of heart rate variability. *Homeost. Health Dis.*, 33, 23-33.

[39] Winchell, R. J. and Hoyt, D. B. (1996) Spectral analysis of heart rate variability in the ICU. *J. Surg. Res.*, 63, 11-16.

[40] Jacobi, J.; Fraser, G. L.; Coursin, D. B.; Riker, R. R.; Fontaine, D.; Wittbrodt, E. T.; Chalfin, D. B.; Masica, M. F.; Bjerke, H. S.; Coplin, W. M.; Crippen, D. W.; Fuchs, B. D.; Kelleher, R. M.; Marik, P. E.; Nasraway, S. A. Jr.; Murray, M. J.; Peruzzi, W. T., and Lumb, D. P. (2002) Clinical practice guidelines for the sustained use of sedatives and analgetics in the critically ill adult. *Crit. Care Med.*, 30, 119-141.

[41] Martin, J.; Bäsell, K.; Bürkle, H.; Hommel, J.; Huth, G.; Kessler, P.; Kretz, F. J.; Putensen, C.; Quintel, M.; Tonner, P.; Tryba, M.; Scholz, J.; Schüttler, J.; Wappler, F., and Spies, C. (2005) Analgesie und Sedierung in der Intensivmedizin – Kurzversion. S2-Leitlinien der Deutschen Gesellschaft für Anästhesiologie und Intensivmedizin (DGAI). *Anästh. Intensivmed.*, 46 (Suppl. 1), S1-S20.

[42] Brullmann, F.; Guidet, B.; Maury, E.; Vassal, T., and Offenstadt, G. (1997) [Analysis of patients´ perception of their stay in a medical intensive care unit.] *Presse Med.*, 26, 1956-1961.

[43] Sjöström, B.; Haljamäe, H.; Dahlgren, L. O., and Lindström, B. (1997) Assessment of postoperative pain: impact of clinical experience and professional role. *Acta Anaesthesiol. Scand.*, 41, 339-344.

[44] Whipple, J. K.; Lewis, K. S.; Quebbeman, E. J.; Wolff, M.; Gottlieb, M. S.; Medicus-Bringa, M.; Harnett, K. R.; Graf, M., and Ausman, R. K. (1995) Analysis of pain management in critically ill patients. *Pharmacotherapy*, 15, 592-599.

[45] Kastrup, M.; von Dossow, V.; Seeling, M.; Ahlborn, R.; Tamarkin, A.; Conroy, P.; Boemke, W.; Wernecke, K. D., and Spies, C. (2009) Key performance indicators in intensive care medicine. A retrospective matched cohort study. *J. Int. Med. Res.*, 37, 1267-1284.

[46] Bowdle, T. A. and Ward, R. J. (1989) Induction of anesthesia with small doses of sufentanil or fentanyl: Dose versus EEG response, speed of onset, and thiopental requirement. *Anesthesiology*, 70, 26-30.

[47] Lin, C. S.; Lu, G.; Ruan, L. Y., and Gu, M. N. (2006) [Patient-controlled intravenous analgesia with sufentanil and fentanyl after thoracotomy: a comparative study.] *Nan Fang Yi Ke Da Xue Xue Bao*, 26, 240-241, 244.

[48] Reves, J. G.; Fragen, R. J.; Vinik, R., and Greenblatt, D. J. (1985) Midazolam: Pharmacology and uses. *Anesthesiology*, 62, 310-324.

[49] Geller, E.; Halpern, P.; Barzelai, E.; Sorkine, P.; Lewis, M. C.; Silbiger, A., and Nevo, Y. (1988) Midazolam infusion and the benzodiazepine antagonist flumazenil for sedation of intensive care patients. *Resuscitation*, 16 (Suppl.), S31-S39.

[50] Patel, S. B. and Kress J. P. (2012) Sedation and analgesia in the mechanically ventilated patient. *Am. J. Respir. Crit. Care Med.*, 185, 486-497.

[51] Komatsu, T.; Singh, P. K.; Kimura, T.; Nishiwaki, K.; Bando, K., and Shimada, Y. (1995) Differential effects of ketamine and midazolam on heart rate variability. *Can. J. Anaesth.*, 42, 1003-1009.

[52] Tsugayasu, R.; Handa, T.; Kaneko, Y., and Ichinohe, T. (2010) Midazolam more effectively suppresses sympathetic activations and reduces stress feelings during mental arithmetic task than propofol. *J. Oral. Maxillofac. Surg.*, 68, 590-596.

[53] Walley, K. R.; Becker, C. J.; Hogan, R. A.; Teplinsky, K., and Wood, L. D. (1988) Progressive hypoxemia limits left ventricular oxygen consumption and contractility. *Circ. Res.*, 63, 849-859.

[54] Baumgartner, C.; Koenighaus, H.; Ebner, J.; Henke, J.; Schuster, T., and Erhardt, W. (2011) Comparison of dipyrone/propofol versus fentanyl /propofol anaesthesia during surgery in rabbits. *Lab. Anim.*, 45, 38-44.

[55] Reddy, P.; Liu, W. S.; Port, D.; Gillmor, S., and Stanley, T. H. (1980) Comparison of haemodynamic effects of anaesthetic doses of alphaprodine and sufentanil in the dog. *Can. Anaesth. Soc. J.*, 27, 345-50.

[56] Kanaya, N.; Zakhary, D. R.; Murray, P. A., and Damron, D. S. (1998) Differential effects of fentanyl and morphine on intracellular Ca^{2+} transients and contraction in rat ventricular myocytes. *Anesthesiology*, 89, 1532-1542.

[57] Bhavsar. R.; Sloth, E.; Folkersen, L.; Greisen, J. R., and Jakobsen, C. J. (2011) Sufentanil preserves hemodynamics and left ventricular function in patients with ischemic heart disease. *Acta Anaesthesiol. Scand.*, 55, 1002-1009.

[58] Leong, K. S.; Mann, P.; Wallymahmed, M.; MacFarlane, I. A., and Wilding, J. P. (1999) Abnormal heart rate variability in adults with growth hormone deficiency. *J. Clin. Endocrin. Metabol.*, 85, 628-633.

[59] Yien, H. W.; Hseu, S. S.; Lee, L. C.; Kuo, T. B.; Lee, T. Y., and Chan, S. H. (1997) Spectral analysis of systemic arterial pressure and heart rate signals as a prognostic tool for the prediction of patient outcome in the intensive care unit. *Crit. Care Med.*, 25, 258-266.

[60] Hadase, M.; Azuma, A.; Zen, K.; Asada, S.; Kawasaki, T.; Kamitani, T.; Kawasaki, S.; Sugihara, H., and Matsubara, H. (2004) Very low frequency power of heart rate variability is a powerful predictor of clinical prognosis in patients with congestive heart failure. *Circ. J.*; 68. 343-347.

[61] Antonelli Incalzi, R.; Corsonello, A.; Trojano, L.; Pedone, C.; Acanfora, D.; Spada, A.; D'Addio, G.; Maestri, R.; Rengo, F., and Rengo, G. (2009) Heart rate variability and drawing impairment in hypoxemic COPD. *Brain. Cogn.*, 70, 163-170.

[62] Kiviniemi, V. J., Haanpää, H., Kantola, J. H., Jauhiainen, J., Vainionpää, V., Alahuhta, S., Tervonen, O. (2005) Midazolam sedation increases fluctuation and synchrony of the resting brain BOLD signal. *Magn. Reson. Imaging*, 23, 531-537.

[63] Ryan, M. L.; Ogilvie, M. P.; Pereira, B. M., Gomez-Rodriguez, J. C.; Manning, R. J.; Vargas, P. A.; Duncan, R. C., and Proctor, K. G. (2011) Heart rate variability is an independent predictor of morbidity and

mortality in hemodynamically stable trauma patients. *J. Trauma*, 70, 1371-1380.

[64] Tateishi, Y.; Oda, S.; Nakamura, M.; Watanabe, K.; Kuwaki, T.; Moriguchi, T., and Hirasawa, H. (2007) Depressed heart rate variability is associated with high IL-6 blood level and decline in the blood pressure in septic patients. *Shock*, 28, 549-553.

[65] Degoute, C. S.; Ray, M. J.; Manchon, M.; Claustrat, B., and Banssillon, V. (1989) Intraoperative glucose infusion and blood lactate: endocrine and metabolic relationships during abdominal surgery. *Anesthesiology*, 71, 355-361.

[66] Moore, P. G.; Quail, A. W.; Cottee, D. B.; McIlveen, S. A., and White, S. W. (2000) Effect of fentanyl on baroreflex control of circumflex coronary conductance. *Clin. Exp. Pharmacol. Physiol.*, 27, 1028-1033.

[67] Tattersall, G. J. and Milsom, W. K. (2009) Hypoxia reduces the hypothalamic thermogenic threshold and thermosensitivity. *J. Physiol.*, 587, 5259–5274.

[68] Reneman, R. S. and Van der Vusse, G. J. (1982) Effect of fentanyl on the myocardial metabolism during ischemia. *Angiology*, 33, 51-63.

[69] Metz, C. and Taeger, K. (2000) [Head-brain injury and cerebral hypoxia. Diagnosis—monitoring—therapy.] *Anaesthesist*, 49, 332-339.

[70] Finney, S. J.; Zekveld, C.; Elia, A., and Evans, T. W. (2003) Glucose control and mortality in critically ill patients. *JAMA*, 290, 2041–2047.

[71] Cheung, N. W.; Li, S.; Ma, G., and Crampton, R. (2008) The relationship between admission blood glucose levels and hospital mortality. *Diabetologia*, 51, 952-955.

[72] Zelihic, E.; Poneleit, B.; Siegmund, T.; Haller, B.; Sayk, F., and Dodt, C. (2014) Hyperglycemia in emergency patients – prevalence and consequences: results of the GLUCEMERGE analysis. *Eur. J. Emerg. Med.*, Sep. 12.

[73] Singer, M. (2007) Mitochondrial function in sepsis: Acute phase versus multiple organ failure. *Crit. Care Med.*, 35, S441-S448.

[74] Talbot, C. R. and Stiffler, D. F. (1991) Effects of hypoxia on acid-base balance, blood gases, catecholamines, and cutaneous ion exchange in the larval tiger salamander (Ambystoma tigrinum). *J. Exp. Zool.*, 257, 299–305.

[75] deZengotita, V. M.; Miller, W. M.; Aunins, J. G., and Zhou, W. (2000) Phosphate feeding improves high-cell-concentration NS0 myeloma culture performance for monoclonal antibody production. *Biotechnol. Bioeng.*, 69, 566-576.

[76] Duewelhenke, N.; Krut, O. and Eysel, P. (2007) Influence of mitochondria and cytotoxicity of different antibiotics administered in high concentrations on primary human osteoblasts and cell lines. *Antimicrob. Agents Chemother.*, 51, 54-63.

[77] Jaiswal, M.; McKeon, K.; Comment, N.; Henderson, J.; Swanson, S.; Plunkett, C.; Nelson, P., and Pop-Busui, R. (2014) Association between impaired cardiovascular autonomic function and hypoglycemia in patients with type 1 diabetes. *Diabetes Care*, 37, 2616-2621.

[78] Kalopita, S.; Liatis, S.; Thomakos, P.; Vlahodimitris, I.; Stathi, C.; Katsilambros, N.; Tentolouris, N., and Makrilakis, K. (2014) Relationship between autonomic nervous system function and continuous interstitial glucose measurement in patients with type 2 diabetes. *J. Diabetes Res.*, 2014, 835392.

[79] Lanspa, M. J.; Dickerson, J.; Morris, A. H.; Orme, J. F.; Holmen, J., and Hirshberg, E. L. (2014) Coefficient of glucose variation is independently associated with mortality in critically ill patients receiving intravenous insulin. *Crit. Care*, 18, R86.

[80] Donati, A.; Damiani, E.; Domizi, R.; Botticelli, L.; Castagnani, R.; Gabbanelli, V.; Nataloni, S.; Carsetti, A.; Scorcella, C.; Adrario, E.; Pelaia, P., and Preiser, J. C. (2014) Glycaemic variability, infections and mortality in a medical-surgical intensive care unit. *Crit. Care Resusc.*, 16, 13-23.

[81] Todi, S. and Bhattacharya, M. (2014) Glycemic variability and outcome in critically ill. *Indian J. Crit. Care Med.*, 18, 285-290.

[82] Tiruvoipati, R.; Chiezey, B.; Lewis, D.; Ong, K.; Villanueva, E.; Haji, K. and Botha, J. (2011) Stress hyperglycemia may not be harmful in critically ill patients with sepsis. *J. Crit. Care*, 27, 153-158.

[83] Christ, B. (2000) Untersuchungen zur Dosierung und Pharmakokinetik von Midazolam bei langzeitsedierten Intensivpatienten. Inaugural-Dissertation, *Justus-Liebig-Universität Gießen*. http://bibd.uni-giessen.de/gdoc/2000/uni/d000093.pdf.

[84] Annane, D.; Trabold, F.; Sharshar, T.; Jarrin, I.; Blanc, A. S.; Raphael, J. C., and Gajdos, P. (1999) Inappropriate sympathetic activation at onset of septic shock. A spectral analysis approach. *Am. J. Respir. Crit. Care Med.*, 160, 458-465.

[85] Hidaka, S.; Kawamoto, M.; Kurita, S., and Yuge, O. (2005) Comparison of the effects of propofol and midazolam on the cardiovascular autonomic nervous system during combined spinal and epidural anesthesia. *J. Clin. Anesth.*, 17, 36-43.

[86] Win, N. N.; Fukuyama, H.; Kohase, H., and Umino, M. (2005) The different effects of intravenous propofol and midazolam sedation on hemodynamic and heart rate variability. *Anesth. Analg.*, 101, 97-102.

[87] Niwa, H.; Tanimoto, A.; Sugimura, M.; Morimoto, Y., and Hanamoto, H. (2006) Cardiovascular effects of epinephrine under sedation with nitrous oxide, propofol, or midazolam. *Oral Surg. Oral Med. Oral Pathol. Oral Radiol. Endod.*, 102, e1-e9.

[88] Buchheit, M.; Richard, R.; Doutreleau, S.; Lonsdorfer-Wolf, E.; Brandenberger, G., and Simon, C. (2004) Effect of acute hypoxia on heart rate variability at rest and during exercise. *Int. J. Sports Med.*, 25, 264-269.

[89] Saito, S.; Tanobe, K.; Yamada, M., and Nishihara, F. (2005) Relationship between arterial oxygen saturation and heart rate variability at high altitudes. *Am. J. Emerg. Med.*, 23, 8-12.

[90] Koelwyn, G. L.; Wong, L. E.; Kennedy, M. D., and Eves, N. D. (2013) The effect of hypoxia and exercise on heart rate variability, immune response, and orthostatic stress. *Scand. J. Med. Sci. Sports*, 23, e1-e8.

In: Septic Shock
Editor: Benedict Graver
ISBN: 978-1-63463-916-3

Chapter III

Angiogenesis-Related Factors and Their Pivotal Role In Septic Shock: A Novel Therapeutic Target and Prognostic Tool

Rolando Martínez, Sergio Vera, Felipe Maira, Matías Libuy, Juan G. Gormaz, and Ramón Rodrigo*

Molecular and Clinical Pharmacology Program,
Institute of Biomedical Sciences, Faculty of Medicine,
University of Chile, Santiago, Chile

Abstract

Endothelial cells are essential elements for vascular homeostasis. Their functions are modulated by several molecules, including angiogenesis-related factors. The latter are not solely involved in

* Corresponding author: Dr. Ramón Rodrigo, Molecular and Clinical Pharmacology Program, Institute of Biomedical Sciences, Faculty of Medicine, University of Chile, Independencia 1027, Santiago, Región Metropolitana, C.P. 8380453, Chile, Phone: +56 2 29786126, Email: rrodrigo@med.uchile.cl

physiological processes such as endothelium maturation and survival, and angiogenesis -a complex process where a new blood vessel is formed from a preexisting one-, but also in pathological conditions, including tumor growth, metastasis and sepsis. Particularly, in severe sepsis the pro-inflammatory state leads to an impairment caused by several mechanisms, resulting into endothelial dysfunction. Angiogenesis-related factors have a pivotal role in the pathophysiological cascade giving rise to this condition, as these molecules contribute to the development of increased capillary permeability, vasoplegia and pro-coagulant and pro-inflammatory states, which could culminate on a septic shock. Recent clinical studies have shown a correlation between the imbalance of the angiogenic growth factors -affecting mainly the angiopoietins and vascular endothelial growth factor pathways- and the poor outcome of patients enduring severe sepsis and septic shock. Different therapies involving the favorable regulation of these angiogenic factors have shown beneficial effects in the pathological events observed in severe sepsis, such as microcirculatory impairment, cardiac fibrosis and hypertrophy, progression towards septic shock and mortality. Therefore, angiogenic growth factors represent a novel prognostic tool in severe sepsis and septic shock. Moreover, these data suggest that angiogenic pathways represent a therapeutic target for future interventions. The design of clinical trials aimed to evaluate the efficacy and safety of anti-angiogenic agents in septic patients is mandatory.

Keywords: Angiogenic factors, septic shock, endothelium, vascular endothelial growth factor, angiopoietins

Abbreviations

AP-1:	Activator protein 1
Ang:	Angiopoietins
ARF:	Angiogenesis-related factors
CLP:	Cecal ligation and puncture
Dll4:	Delta-like ligand 4
Egfl7:	Epidermal growth factor-like protein 7
eNOS:	Endothelial nitric oxide synthase
FGF:	Fibroblast growth factor
HIF-α:	Hypoxia inducing factor alpha
ICAM-1:	Intercellular adhesion molecule 1
IL:	Interleukine
iNOS:	Inducible nitric oxide synthase

LPS:	Lipopolysaccharide
NF-κB:	Nuclear factor kappa B
NO:	Nitric oxide
NOS:	Nitric oxide synthase
PAI-1:	Plasminogen activator inhibitor-1
PAMPs:	Pathogen-associated molecular patterns
PDGF:	Platelet-derived growth factor
PlGF:	Placental growth factor
RhoA:	Ras homolog gene family member A
RNS:	Reactive nitrogen species
ROS:	Reactive oxygen species
sFlt-1	soluble form of the VEGFR-1
TGF- β:	Transforming growth factor-beta
Tie	tyrosine kinase receptor
TLR:	Toll-like receptor
TNF- α:	Tumor necrosis factor-alpha
VCAM-1:	Vascular adhesion molecule 1
VE-cadherin:	Vascular endothelial cadherin
VEGF:	Vascular endothelial growth factor

Introduction

Angiogenesis is a dynamic process responsible for the formation of new vascular structures from preexisting vessels. It accounts for the growth and remodeling of the primitive vascular network of organs. Several physiological factors contribute to the maintenance of a balance between pro-angiogenic and angiostatic factors. These factors play a key role in regulating endothelial cell function, a cell type implicated in complex disease processes including modulation of vascular tone, thrombosis, inflammatory responses and new vessel formation. Endothelial cells function is substantial for cardiovascular integrity, on both macro and microcirculatory levels. Specifically on sepsis, endothelial dysfunction drives to important microvascular changes that affect organ function, and also leads to vasoplegia and tissue edema with the subsequent hypotension and hypovolemia; culminating on septic shock. The last is a severe complication of sepsis that increases mortality rate even with the current manages of the international guidelines. Therefore, the design of new therapeutic strategies is mandatory. On this line, angiogenesis-related factors (ARF) seem to be strongly involved in the production of endothelial alterations, thus opening a new opportunity for diagnosis and treatment. At present, there are several biomarkers accounting for the functional impairment in sepsis and for its progression towards septic shock. The objective of this chapter is to give an insight on the pathophysiological mechanisms involved in endothelial dysfunction and their relation to ARF balanced alterations induced on septic patients, and to discuss the promising results of pre-clinical studies using ARF molecules.

1. Angiogenesis-Related Factors

Angiogenic related factors are molecules that regulate the complex process known as angiogenesis, corresponding to the development of new blood vessels out of existing ones in physiological, compensatory or even pathological conditions [1], including tumor vascularization, diabetic retinopathy, psoriasis, and rheumatoid arthritis, among others [2]. Angiogenesis is a continuous process that can be divided into three major steps: I. destabilization phase; II. proliferation and migration phase; III. maturation phase. In destabilization phase, endothelial cells become activated; loosen their contact with each other and their environment leading to increased vascular permeability, deposition of fibrin into the extra-vascular space, vessel wall disassembly and base membrane degradation. During the proliferation and migration phase, the endothelial cells migrate on and into the fibrin scaffold towards the angiogenic stimulus and proliferate, aligning and thus forming a capillary lumen. Finally, in the maturation phase, endothelial cells proliferation and migration are inhibited and the junctional complexes and base membrane are assembled, thus stabilizing the newly formed blood vessel [2]. ARF might be classified in two categories: pro-angiogenic growth factors -such as vascular endothelial growth factor (VEGF), angiopoietins (Ang), fibroblast growth factor, among others- [3] and anti-angiogenic factors -including endostatin, thrombospondin, angiostatin and platelet factor 4- [4]. These factors are in a delicate balance; however under certain stimuli this equilibrium is disrupted leading to angiogenesis or vascular degeneration by increased concentration of pro-angiogenic or anti-angiogenic factors respectively (Table 1).

Table 1. Factors that promote and inhibit angiogenesis

Pro-angiogenic factors	Function in angiogenesis	References	Anti-angiogenic factors	Function in angiogenesis	References
Ang-1, Ang-2	Fundamental role in the maintenance of vessel integrity.	5; 6	Angioarrestin	Inhibits various angiogenic processes through its effect on both the induction and resolution phases of the angiogenic cascade	8
Angiogenin	Migration, proliferation and tube formation.	7	Angiostatin	Inhibit endothelial cell proliferation, endothelial migration and/or promote endothelial apoptosis	19
ARP 1, ARP 2	Endothelial sprouting	8	Anti-thrombin III	Inhibition of FGF-2 and VEGF-induced proliferation of endothelial cells	20
CDT6	Pro-angiogenic activity in the cornea	9; 10	Canstatin, endostatin, prolactin	Affect the basement membrane and extra-cellular matrix	2
Ephrins	Vascular development during embryogenesis and in adult angiogenesis	11; 12	2-Methoxyestradiol	Decreases migration, invasion and tubule formation	21
FGF	Modulation of endothelial cell proliferation, migration, protease production, integrin and cadherin receptor expression, and intercellular gap-junction communication	13; 14	IFN-α,β,χ	Prevent proliferation, migration and differentiation of endothelial cells	22; 23
HGF, TP, NPY	Plateled-derived regulators, affecting endothelial cells proliferation and migration	2; 15; 16	IL-4, IL-12, IL-18	Induce chemokins that exerts antiangiogenic effects	24; 25

Table 1. (Continued)

Pro-angiogenic factors	Function in angiogenesis	References	Anti-angiogenic factors	Function in angiogenesis	References
PDGF, EGF, TGFβ	Cellular proliferation and migration	2	PEDF	Promotes proapoptotic mechanisms, prevents cell migration, inhibits endothelial tube formation and vessel sprouting	26
PGAR	Endothelial survival factor	2	Plasminogen activator inhibitor	Inhibits tPA and uPA	27
TF, thrombin, uPA, tPA, plasmin, MMPs, chymases, heparanases	Affect the basement membrane and extra-cellular matrix	2	Platelet factor 4	Inhibits binding of endothelial growth factors	2
TNF-α	Stimulates proliferation, migration/invasion, and the formation of new blood vessels by endothelial cells	17	TSP-1	Inhibit endothelial cell proliferation, migration and tube formation	28
VEGF	Mediates vascular permeability, endothelial proliferation, migration and survival	2; 18; 1			

Ang: Angiopoietin; ARP: Angiopoietin-Related Protein; CDT6: Cornea-Derived Transcript 6; EGF: Epidermal Growth Factor; FGF: Fibroblast Growth Factor; HGF: Hepatocyte Growth Factor; IFN: Interferon; IL: Interleukin; MMPs: matrix metalloproteases; NPY: Neuropeptide Y; PDGF: Platelet-Derived Growth Factor; PEDF: Pigment-Epithelium Derived Factor; PGAR: Peroxisome proliferator-activated receptor γ, Angiopoietin-Related; TF: Tissue Factor; TGF: Transforming Growth Factor; TNF-α: Tumor Necrosis Factor; TP: Thymidine Phosphorylase; tPA: tissue Plasminogen Activator; TSP-1: Thrombospondin 1; uPA: urokinase-type Plasminogen Activator; VEGF: Vascular Endothelial Growth Factor

Furthermore, on quiescent endothelial cells, autocrine and paracrine actions of pro-angiogenic growth factors act as cell-survival signals, which are essential for endothelial function and structural integrity; this is accomplished by inhibition of inflammation and apoptosis, suppression of vascular leakage, and regulation of intercellular junction, among other effects [29, 30]. Thus the correct balance of ARF is crucial to maintain the cardiovascular homeostasis [31]. In the mechanisms that account for the development of sepsis and its complications, imbalance of VEGF and angiopoietin pathways are especially important. Therefore, their roles in the physiology and pathophysiology of cardiovascular homeostasis will be reviewed in more detail.

1.1. VEGF Superfamily

Vascular endothelial growth factor is an endothelial cell specific mitogen that was first identified as a tumor-produced vascular permeability factor, but it is also essential for angiogenesis, playing a crucial role in wound healing [32]. It is a family of six molecules: VEGF-A (or VEGF), placental growth factor (PlGF), VEGF-B, VEGF-C, VEGF-D, and orf virus VEGF (VEGF-E), in which every single member plays an irreplaceable role in the development of the vascular system of the embryo [34].

There are at least eight isoforms of the VEGF-A molecule that are determined by the length of amino acids in its chain as consequence of the alternative splicing of the VEGF-A gene. Only the shorter one (VEGF121) is soluble, and promotes vessel enlargement, whereas matrix-bound isoforms stimulate branching [3; 34]. The predominant isoform VEGF165 binds to VEGFR-1, VEGFR-2, Neuropilin-1 and Neuropilin-2 [2]. The binding of VEGF to VEGFR-1 and VEGFR-2 results in activation of specific pathways that regulates proliferation, migration and survival of vascular endothelial cells, thus resulting in angiogenesis, while VEGF-C and D binds to VEGFR-3 to regulate proliferation, migration and survival of lymphatic endothelial cells. On other hand, Neuropilin 1 and 2 function as indirect angiogenic factors when activated by VEGF. This activation induces endothelial cell migration and sprouting [35].

It is important to notice that the principal functions originated by VEGF are consequence of VEGFR-2 binding, which triggers the PI3 kinase-AKT pathway. In low oxygen conditions the Hypoxia-Inducing Factor alpha (HIF-α) -a molecule that appears in the context of hypoxia and oxidative stress-, which is permanently being degraded in normoxemic conditions, induces the translocation of transcriptional factors from the cytoplasm into the nucleus. This results in the activation of nuclear factor kappa B (NF-κB) pathway triggering the production of cytokines, interleukins, and VEGF, among other growth factors, and thus increasing the activation of VEGFR-2. There are many other molecules that regulate the levels of VEGF in the blood, being Endothelin-1, Angiotensin-II, and matrix metalloproteinase the main ones [35]. To maintain the vascular homeostasis, a balance between vascular vasoconstrictor and vasodilator factors is needed. VEGF, among other molecules, regulates this balance by inhibiting endothelin, a potent vasoconstrictor. Similarly, nitric oxide (NO), which production is induced by VEGF, also inhibits endothelin [35]. Moreover, VEGF is fundamental in maintaining the endothelial cell function. This is accomplished due to mitogenic and anti-apoptotic effect vascular endothelial cells, which is induced by the activation of the PI3-AKT pathway [36, 37].

The vascular tone is mediated mainly by both the levels of intracellular calcium ions and the synthesis and release of NO. Both of these parameters are regulated by the action of VEGF-VEGFR2, which induce vasodilatation by increasing phospholipase C, protein kinase C and inositol 1,4,5 triphosphate activity, resulting in decreased intracellular calcium ions and increased synthesis and release of NO [38].

In response to several agents often associated with sepsis, such as gram-negative bacterial LPS, gram-positive bacterial components, and Tumor necrosis factor-α (TNF-α), VEGF production or secretion of the intracellular pool is increased [32]. VEGF also plays a fundamental role in increasing vascular density in situations of hypoxia and ischemic cardiomyopathy [39]. The formation of new blood vessels is regularized by the production of HIF-α, which functions include induction of cytokine release, as previously mentioned. These molecules increase vascular permeability which leads to leakage of plasma proteins [40].

1.2. Angiopoietins Family

Angiopoietin and its specific tyrosine kinase receptor (Tie) is a molecular system that acts controlling the endothelial cell survival and the vascular maturation. This family includes four ligands: Angiopoietin-1 (Ang-1), Angiopoietin-2 (Ang-2), Angiopoietin-3/4 (Ang-3/4), and two corresponding tyrosine kinase receptors (Tie-1 and Tie-2). The main molecules of this family involved in the vascular regulation and maturation are Ang-1 and Ang-2, and their antagonist actions over Tie-2. While Ang-1 acts in a paracrine agonist manner activating Tie-2, Ang-2 acts in an autocrine antagonist way when binding to the same receptor [41]. Even though Tie-1 remains an orphan receptor without any specific ligand, gene targeting studies have revealed that both Tie-1 and Tie-2 are essential for vascular maturation. In Tie-1 null embryos, angiogenesis is not perturbed, yet vessels lose their integrity, leading to widespread edema, hemorrhage and death [42]. The genetic experiments suggest that Tie-1 plays important roles during endothelial cell differentiation and in the regulation of vessel integrity [41]. Studies with Tie-2 deficient mouse embryos showed that they died in earlier stages of the embryogenesis due to vessel remodeling defects in the plexus of the yolk sac and the brain, and severe heart defects. The quality of the resulting vessels was diminished, with fewer branches, reduced pericyte coverage and poor organization. Tie-2 has also shown a critical role in hematopoiesis [41]. On the other hand, Ang-1 is a single non-redundant agonist of Tie-2 required for endothelial cell survival and proliferation and for vessel maturation. It has been seen that double-transgenic mice expressing both Ang-1 and VEGF-A in the skin show more and enlarged blood vessels. From these results it is concluded that Ang-1 and VEGF regulate angiogenesis at distinct levels, with VEGF inducing vessel sprouting and growth and Ang-1 mediating vessel remodeling and maturation [42]. It may be possible that the Ang-1/Tie-2 signals also regulates the expression of other factors, such as Delta-like ligand 4 (Dll4), a protein that binds Notch ,a highly conserved cell signaling system, resulting in signals that produces a negative regulatory effects on angiogenesis, and specially diminishing vascular sprouting. Related to this, the signaling produced by Dll4/Notch, augmented by Ang-1/Tie-2 signaling, induces the extracellular deposition of collagen type IV, a major component of the basement membrane, during endothelial cell tube formation and thereby promoting vascular stabilization [44]. Furthermore, it has been shown that Ang-2 levels are elevated in several diseases associated with vascular dysfunction, including inflammatory disorders such as sepsis [44]. Ang-2-defficient mice are born normally and can develop to adulthood; however, they will have developed multiple vascular defects when reaching this stage. When functioning as an Ang-1 antagonist, Ang-2 promotes the dissociation of pericytes from pre-existing vessels and increases vascular permeability [45]. This allows the output of cytokines, proteases, and angiogenic myeloid cells, that in the presence of growth factors, such as VEGF A, allow a robust angiogenic response. The endothelial cell of unstable vessels lacking pericytes have different fates: they die in the absence of VEGF, but migrate or proliferate in the presence of VEGF depending on whether they are located at the sprouting tip or the stalk of a newly forming blood vessel [46].

High levels of Ang-2, functioning as an Ang-1 antagonist, prevent pericyte recruitment to the newly formed vessel sprouts and help to maintain the unstable nature of endothelial cell. The proliferation and migration of endothelial cell will result in an endothelial cell network that cannot conduct blood flow unless a vessel lumen is formed. In proliferating tissues, epidermal growth factor-like protein 7 (Egfl-7) is highly expressed, and binds to blood vessel extracellular matrix promoting the formation of endothelial tubes with a lumen. In contrast, Transforming Growth Factor β (TGF-β), a protein that controls proliferation and cellular differentiation in most cells, represses vascular tube formation and pericyte recruitment [47]. Ang-1 can overcome TGF-β-mediated inhibition of VEGF-induced endothelial cell tube formation, whereas Ang-2 promotes this inhibitory effect of TGF-β [48].

2. Septic Shock Pathophysiology and ARF

Sepsis, the systemic inflammatory response due to a microbial infection, is an extensive clinical problem with significant mortality and economic burden [49], moreover it leads to several complications with increased mortality rates, such as severe sepsis (25-30%) and septic shock (40-70%) [50]. Severe sepsis involves sepsis plus sepsis-induced organ dysfunction or tissue hypoperfusion, which are defined by several laboratory criteria. Septic shock is sepsis-induced hypotension (systolic blood pressure < 90 mmHg or mean arterial pressure < 70 mmHg in the absence of other causes of hypotension), elevated lactate or oliguria persisting despite adequate fluid resuscitation [50] These last alterations are due to profound hemodynamic alterations associated with organ dysfunction, including hypovolemia, decrease in vascular tone and myocardial depression [51].

2.1. Sepsis Progression Towards Septic Shock

On sepsis, the pathogen-associated molecular patterns (PAMPs) of the infecting bacteria -mainly lipopolysaccharides and exotoxins [52] -are recognized by special cell receptors called "Pattern recognition receptors" - TLR, NOD- leading to an activation of the NF-κB transcriptional factor and activator protein 1 (AP-1). NF-κB and AP-1, among other effects, increases the secretion of pro-inflammatory cytokines (TNF-α, IL-1, IL-2, IL-6, IL-8, IFNγ) [53], producing a hyper-inflammatory response that exceeds the boundaries of local environment generating a systemic reaction.

Pro-inflammatory cytokines activate endothelial cells and leukocytes. Activated endothelium increases its permeability, up-regulates adhesion molecules -ICAM-1 and VCAM-1-, and leans toward a procoagulant state; this leads to tissue edema, fibrin deposition and leukocytes infiltration [54]. Activated leukocytes extravasate into surrounding tissues and increase their production of proteases, cytotoxic enzymes, reactive oxygen species (ROS), -such as H_2O_2, HClO and O_2^-- and reactive nitrogen species (RNS) -NO and $ONOO^-$-[54] The increased generation of these reactive species leads to a state known as oxidative stress -a harmful condition that causes biological damage and it is produced when pro-oxidant molecules exceed the protective antioxidant mechanism of the cell [55]-, which contributes to microvascular and tissue damage [54]. In this context, ROS and RNS have been associated with an amplification of the pro inflammatory state of sepsis in the surrounding tissues. This might be explained by the capacity of some reactive species to increase the activity of the transcription factors NF-κB and AP1 [56]. Therefore, the production of ROS/RNS is increased on sepsis and contributes to the pro-inflammatory state, thus generating a positive feedback system.

2.2. Endothelial and Microvascular Dysfunction

The endothelium is essential for vascular homeostasis, due to its role in the modulation of vasomotor tone, blood fluidity, cellular and nutrient trafficking; local balance in pro-inflammatory and anti-inflammatory mediators, angiogenesis and programmed cell death, among other processes [57]. Moreover the endothelium plays a pivotal role in the normal function of the microcirculation [58].

The primary role of the microcirculation is to provide optimal exchange of gases, nutrients and metabolites between the blood and surrounding tissues [59], therefore, cell survival and an adequate organ function depends on adequate microvascular function [60]. A second important role of the microvascular bed is to limit large fluctuations in hydrostatic pressure within the thin-walled capillaries. This is achieved at the level of arterioles through regulation of vascular tone, making the microvasculature an important site for the regulation of local and overall peripheral resistance and hence blood pressure [61].

In a sepsis state, as a consequence of the increase of cytokines and reactive species, the normal functioning of the endothelial cells is impaired, triggering apoptosis and endothelial dysfunction [62], thus, amplifying the pro-coagulant and pro-inflammatory states of sepsis, increasing endothelial permeability and altering the vasomotor response [54]. These alterations seem to be ubiquitous in all sepsis animal models [63, 64] and it has been observed in human tissues as well [65] unchaining a global microcirculatory failure [66]. Accordingly, tissue edema, fibrin deposition, blood clotting, heterogeneous capillary perfusion and reduced capacity for tissue oxygen extraction are produced, contributing to the decline on organ function associated with sepsis [67].

As sepsis progresses these alterations are transversely accentuated, affecting organ function throughout the economy, eventually producing severe sepsis and septic shock. Among the pathophysiological processes involved in the genesis of these complications -cardiovascular dysfunction, produced mainly by depressed myocardial function and microcirculatory alterations and mitochondrial dysfunction- ARF are strongly involved on the generation and maintenance of the microcirculatory changes related to septic shock.

2.3. ARF Pathways Response to Septic State and Their Role on Inflammation

Sepsis is associated to high circulating levels of VEGF on human studies [32]. Several stimuli often associated with sepsis increases VEGF production or secretion -by endothelial cells, vascular smooth cells, leukocytes and platelets-, including: hypoxia, NO, blood clotting and bacterial endotoxin [68]. Furthermore, on a murine LPS-injection model, pro-inflammatory cytokines had been associated with increased VEGF release by leukocytes [69] and exogenous administration of VEGF enhanced the increase in TNF-α and IL-1 on a murine LPS-injection model [70]. In addition, an increased activity of the NF-κB has been attributed to VEGF [71].

In human endotoxemia and sepsis, circulating Ang-1 levels remain unchanged, or even decrease, whereas Ang-2 is rapidly released by the activated endothelium. Hence, the balance between circulating Ang-1 and Ang-2 is shifted in favor of the more dynamic player Ang-2, thus decreasing Tie-2 activity [18, 72]. Ang-2 is stored on Weibel-Palade bodies and is rapidly released from endothelial vesicles, upon different inflammatory stimuli (e.g., TNF-α, LPS, hypoxia), mediated by an increase on calcium influx [73]. Therefore, secretion of both VEGF and Ang-2 are significantly increased on septic patients. Moreover, their implications on the increase inflammatory phenotype of endothelial cells -with increased proinflammatory cytokines secretion, increased adhesion molecules, among other effect- might generate a positive feedback system.

2.4. ARF Effects in Microcirculatory Alteration on Septic Shock

Mechanical forces are profoundly modified during distributive shocks like septic shock, characterized by a major hypovolemia and intense vasoplegia [54]. Endothelial dysfunction is known to be a critical element in the pathogenesis of these phenomena, mainly by the development of microcirculatory dysfunction [67, 74], characterized by: loss of the endothelial glycocalyx, which covers the endothelium and forms an important barrier and transduction system; increased microvascular permeability with capillary leakage, edema formation; decreased red blood cells deformability, with secondary capillary plugging; and impaired arteriolar smooth muscle cell tone and reactivity, among other effects [74]. These microcirculatory alteration may appear without any hemodynamic global effect -absence of hypotension- [75], i.e an adequate blood pressure and normal oxygen saturation do not necessarily correlate with an adequate oxygen distribution on tissues level or correct oxygen utilization by cells, -which might explain the poor results on septic shock survival even with current therapies [76, 77, 78]. Moreover, an association has been proven between the severity of microcirculatory dysfunction with development of multiple organ dysfunction syndrome [74, 79] and poor outcome of septic patients [74, 80].

2.4.1. Sepsis-Induced Vascular Hyporeactivity

Vascular hyporeactivity (vasoplegia) is a form of vasodilatory shock, characterized by markedly low systemic pressure and systemic vascular resistance –despite adequate fluid resuscitation and adrenergic vasopressor administration-, impairment of vascular reactivity to vasopressor agents -such as catecholamine, vasopressin, angiotensin II- and imbalance between the vasoconstrictor and vasodilator tone; leading to a heterogeneous perfusion [81, 82]. The mechanisms responsible for these phenomena seem to be a combination of endothelial injury, arginine-vasopressin system dysfunction, release of other vasodilatory inflammatory mediators –such as chemokines, NO and VEGF-, and muscle hyperpolarization [81]. Among them, NO imbalance it is specially related to ARF. Physiologically, NO is produced in picomolar concentrations from L-arginine by a constitutively enzyme expressed on endothelial cells, the endothelial nitric oxide synthase (eNOS) [83]. NO diffuses into the underlying vascular smooth muscle and induces vasorelaxation via stimulation of soluble guanylate cyclase and resulting in an increased production of cGMP [84, 85]. Additionally, in sepsis conditions, NO production is dramatically increased, principally by the augmented expression of the inducible nitric oxide synthase (iNOS) -stimulated mainly by pro-inflammatory cytokines [86]-, thus contributing to hypotension and vascular hyporeactivity. Notwithstanding, NO synthase (NOS) inhibitors increased mortality on septic patients, despite positive effects on blood pressure and vascular resistance [87], this is probably caused by the suppression of eNOS-derived NO production, which is essential for endothelial function [88]. On this line, VEGF leads to increase activity of NOS by increasing in intracellular calcium; furthermore induces the prostacyclin release pathway via activation of phospholipase A_2 activity [89]. Thus the increased levels of VEGF seen on severe sepsis might contribute to the vasoplegia.

2.4.2. Loss of Endothelial Barrier Function Induced by Sepsis

In sepsis the endothelial barrier function is altered, mainly by alterations on their intercellular junctions, endothelial cell contraction and disruption in their glycocalyx integrity; leading to fluid leakage from the intravascular space with subsequent edema and increased rolling and adhesion of leukocytes [54]. The loss of the integrity of endothelial junctions due to deregulation of its components is initiated by pro-inflammatory cytokines, chemokines, and ARF. They stimulate the phosphorylation of the major component of this intercellular interaction, the vascular endothelial cadherin (VE-cadherin), producing its internalization [90]. Endothelial cell contraction is mediated by cytoskeleton alterations. In inflammatory pathologies the actin filaments –main structural components of the cytoskeleton- structure is affected by the increased activity of the Ras homolog gene family member A (RhoA), thus leading to cell contraction and consequent gap formation [91]. Finally, the glycocalyx is a thin layer of glucosaminoglycans that covers the endothelial surface. Sepsis stimulates the shedding of the glycocalyx, evidenced on a markedly decreased size -according to transmission electron microscopy measurements- and increased levels of byproducts of its degradation in the blood. This contributes to increased vascular permeability, by a reduced sieve function, and by rearranging cytoskeletal proteins and altering intercellular junctions [92, 93]. Several studies suggest a strong involvement of the Ang-2/Ang-1 increased ratio on endothelial barrier disruption. The excess of systemic Ang-1 plasma levels improved mortality rate and hemodynamic function in mice models of endotoxic shock [94] and the excess of systemic Ang-2 provoked pulmonary leak and congestion in healthy adult mice [95]. A possible explanation is that the increased Ang-2/Ang-1 ratio augments the RhoA activity, altering the cytoskeleton integrity [96], and inhibition Ang-1-induced changes in microvascular glycocalyx –increased depth and density- [97].

On the other hand VEGF seems to have an important role on these pathophysiological phenomena as well. VEGF is 50,000 times more potent than histamine on increasing vascular permeability and is a potent inducer of tissue edema [98]. This process is mediated by stimulating calcium influx into endothelial cells [99], leading to cytoskeletal reorganization (through myosin-light-chain-dependent contraction) and the disassembly of VE-cadherin at the adherens junctions [100]. Furthermore, high levels of VEGF have been associated with increased glucosaminoglycans shedding; another possible mechanism for VEGF induced hyperpermeability.

3. ARF As Biomarkers of Septic Shock

A biomarker is a molecule in a biological sample, which is measurable in an objective, systematic and precise way, whose levels are indicators of a process it is normal or abnormal, and are used to monitor response to treatment [101]. The most important factors that characterize the ideal biomarker are the sensitivity, specificity, and predictive value [102]. In sepsis, endothelial activation and dysfunction are critical determinants of the host response and represent an explanation for the complex sepsis pathophysiology [27]. Therefore, biomarkers reflecting the state of endothelial cells might be useful in the tracking of sepsis [103, 104].

Different studies have showed that plasma VEGF levels from patients with septic shock are decreased and associated with disease severity (organ dysfunction and unfavorable outcome) [18, 105, 106, 107], in contrast to higher levels in sepsis and at onset of severe sepsis [107]. The soluble form of the VEGFR-1 (sFlt-1), a critical regulator of circulating VEGF bioavailability [108], has been shown to be strongly prognostic in sepsis [109]. It has been described that sFlt-1 levels are higher in septic shock patients, being an independent predictive factor for mortality and the presence of concomitant multiorgan dysfunction [110, 111, 112]. This could be explained by several hypotheses: (i) sFlt-1 levels reflect the vigor of the anti-inflammatory response in sepsis, (ii) elevated sFlt-1 levels may cause immune depression by interfering with sFlt-1 mediated signaling in monocytes, and (iii) sFlt-1 may interfere with endothelial repair by inhibiting VEGF signaling in endothelial cells [79].

Ang-1 and Ang-2 are two of the most widely studied biomarkers of endothelial activation/dysfunction in infectious diseases [113]. As previously described, angiopoietins are endothelial-derived vascular growth factors that play opposing roles during sepsis [114]. Several studies have documented that in severe sepsis and septic shock, Ang-2 levels are higher, and Ang-1 levels are lower [18, 106, 115, 116, 117, 118]. It has also been reported that Ang-1 is independently associated with mortality [18, 27], remaining as a significant predictor of outcome [119], whereas Ang-2 plays a pivotal role in the development of organ dysfunction, thus leading to a poor outcome [115, 118]. Angiopoietins seem to be of interest as prognostic severe sepsis biomarkers of disease severity and patient outcome [120]. Ang-2 might present a reliable marker reflecting the direct status of the endothelium that correlates with sepsis severity and outcome, whereas Ang-1 levels might have a high predictive outcome value, when determined at admission to the ICU [27]. Other angiogenic factors have been documented, such as fibroblast growth factor (FGF), platelet-derived growth factor (PDGF), and plasminogen activator inhibitor-1 (PAI-1). Lower plasma FGF and PDGF concentrations were associated with an unfavorable outcome in children with severe bacterial infection [2, 18].

Currently, there is much enthusiasm and interest in the clinical utility of sepsis biomarkers [121]. However, this utility is limited by lacks of standardization in analytical assays, of data regarding receiver operating characteristics and of validation [122].

4. ARF As Potential Therapeutic Tools

Current management of septic shock focuses in an adequate fluid resuscitation, an appropriate and early antibiotic therapy, and a close monitoring of hemodynamic conditions, using vasopressors agents if necessary [50]. However, although this treatment has been effective, morbidity and mortality still remains elevated. As described before, this is probably by the incapacity of this treatment to correct the microcirculatory alterations associated with septic shock, thus being unable to ensure a correct delivery of oxygen to the tissues. Therefore, as ARF pathways are closely related to microvascular alterations, molecules that correct the imbalance of these factors might improve treatment efficacy and hence increase survival on patients with septic shock. One of the strategies to accomplish the recovery of the normal balance of ARF pathways has been the use of molecules that diminish the activity of VEGF. On this line, the anti-VEGF antibody, Bevacizumab, was used in lethal murine models of sepsis -cecal ligation and puncture (CLP), and lipopolysaccharide (LPS) injection-, resulting in a decreased expression of pro-inflammatory cytokines and decreased permeability on lungs, spleen and kidneys.

The effect of Bevacizumab in mortality showed interesting results: at a low concentration the survival rate was significantly improved, but at higher doses no difference was achieved. The effect of the treatment remained even when it was applied with 6 hours of delay [123]. In addition, sFlt-1 has been used. This soluble form lacks the transmembrane and cytoplasmic domains but retains the ability to bind to its ligands and thus functions as a dominant negative inhibitor of VEGF [124]. Treatment with sFlt-1, on a lethal LPS injection and CLP-induced sepsis model, decreased levels of pro-inflammatory cytokines (TNF-α and IL-1), diminish recruitment of inflammatory cells into the peritoneal cavity and also significantly improved survival [70].

Another strategy used is the restoration of the ratio Ang-2/Ang-1, towards higher levels of Tie2 activity. Therefore, Vasculotide, a novel polyethylene glycol (PEG)-clustered Tie2 agonist peptide, was used on a CLP murine model. The results of this study showed decreased capillary leakage, ameliorated leukocytes transmigration and enhanced survival. The latter effect was more pronounced when the molecule was administered before surgery; however, also positive results were obtained by inoculating the drug two hours later [125]. Moreover, a recombinant form of Ang-1 (rhAng-1) significantly protected against a variety of sepsis-associated organ dysfunctions and improved survival time on a CLP murine model [126]. Finally, the treatment with Ang-2 antibody, on a LPS murine model, attenuated hemodynamic alterations and significantly reduced the mortality rate [127].

Conclusion

Cumulated evidence accounts for a key role of ARF in the mechanism of vascular alterations occurring in septic shock. Available biomarkers could provide valuable data about the contribution of pathological processes, such as inflammation, oxidative stress and endothelial dysfunction, all of them closely related to angiogenesis. Therefore, the paradigm presented on this chapter strongly suggests that angiogenesis-related pathways represent a novel therapeutic target for future interventions. No clinical studies have been published yet using these novel therapies on septic shock patients. Whether these treatments are or are not useful in human sepsis remains as an open question. Therefore the design clinical trials aimed to evaluate the efficacy and safety of anti-angiogenic agents in septic patients is mandatory.

References

[1] Rosen LS. Clinical experience with angiogenesis signaling inhibitors: focus on vascular endothelial growth factor (VEGF) blockers. *Cancer Control,* 2002; 9 (2 Suppl):36-44.

[2] Bouïs D, Kusumanto Y, Meijer C, Mulder NH, Hospers GA. A review on pro- and anti-angiogenic factors as targets of clinical intervention. *Pharmacol. Res.,* 2006; 53 (2):89-103.

[3] Carmeliet P, Jain RK. Molecular mechanisms and clinical applications of angiogenesis. *Nature,* 2011; 473 (7347):298-307.

[4] Ribatti D. Endogenous inhibitors of angiogenesis: a historical review. *Leuk Res.,* 2009; 33 (5):638-44.

[5] Lee J1, Park DY, Park do Y, Park I, Chang W, Nakaoka Y, Komuro I, Yoo OJ, Koh GY. Angiopoietin-1 suppresses choroidal neovascularization and vascular leakage. *Invest Ophthalmol Vis Sci.,* 2014; 55:2191-9.

[6] Koh GY. Orchestral actions of angiopoietin-1 in vascular regeneration. *Trends Mol. Med.,* 2013; 19 (1):31-9.

[7] Yuan Y, Wanga F, Liub X-H, Gong D, Cheng H, Huang S. Angiogenin is involved in lung adenocarcinoma cell proliferation and angiogenesis. *Lung Cancer,* 2009; 66 (1): 28–36.

[8] Dhanabal M, Jeffers M, LaRochelle WJ, Lichenstein HS. Angioarrestin: A unique angiopoietin-related protein with anti-angiogenic properties. *Biochem. Biophys Res Commun,* 2005; 333 (2):308-15.

[9] Liu Y, Paradis H, Gendron RL, Choi DW, Chapon P. AngX/CDT6 a novel fibrinogen/angiopoietin-like factor that enhances angiogenesis in vivo. *Invest. Ophtalmol. Vis. Sci.,* 2001; 42 (4):478.

[10] Peek R, Kammerer RA, Frank S, Otte I, Westphal JR. The angiopoietin-like factor cornea-derived transcript 6 is a putative morphogen for human cornea. *J. Biol. Chem.,* 2001; 277 (1):686–93.

[11] Cheng N, Brantley D, Chen J. The ephrins and Eph receptors in angiogenesis. *Cytokine Growth Factor Rev.,* 2002; 13 (1):75-85.

[12] Kuijper S1, Turner CJ, Adams RH. Regulation of angiogenesis by Eph-ephrin interactions. *Trends Cardiovasc. Med.,* 2007; 17 (5):145-51.

[13] Cross MJ, Claesson-Welsh L. FGF and VEGF function in angiogenesis: signalling pathways, biological responses and therapeutic inhibition. *Trends Pharmacol. Sci.,* 2001; 22 (4):201-7.

[14] Presta M, Dell'Era P, Mitola S, Moroni E, Ronca R, Rusnati M. Fibroblast growth factor/fibroblast growth factor receptor system in angiogenesis. *Cytokine Growth Factor Rev.,* 2005; 16 (2):159-78.

[15] Ieda Y, Fujita J, Ieda M, Yagi T, Kawadac H, Andoc K, et al. G-CSF and HGF: Combination of vasculogenesis and angiogenesis synergistically improves recovery in murine hind limb ischemia. *J. Mol. Cell Cardiol.,* 2007; 42 (3):540-8.

[16] Miyatani T, Kurita N, Utsunomiya T, Iwata T, Nishioka M, Yoshikawa K, et al. Platelet-derived endothelial cell growth factor/thymidine phosphorylase inhibitor augments radiotherapeutic efficacy in experimental colorectal cancer. *Cancer Lett.,* 2012; 318 (2):199–205.

[17] Yang HL, Chang HC, Lin SW, Senthil Kumar KJ, Liao CH, Wang HM, et al. Antrodia salmonea inhibits TNF-α-induced angiogenesis and atherogenesis in human endothelial cells through the down-regulation of NF-κB and up-regulation of Nrf2 signaling pathways. *J. Ethnopharmacol.,* 2014; 151 (1):394-406.

[18] Mankhambo LA, Banda DL; IPD Study Group, Jeffers G, White SA, Balmer P, Nkhoma S, Phiri H, Molyneux EM, Hart CA, Molyneux ME, Heyderman RS, Carrol ED. The role of angiogenic factors in predicting clinical outcome in severe bacterial infection in Malawian children. *Crit. Care,* 2010;14(3):R91.

[19] Radziwon Balicka A, Ramer C, de la Rosa C, Zielnik-Drabik B, Jurasz P. Angiostatin inhibits endothelial MMP-2 and MMP-14 expression: A

hypoxia specific mechanism of action. *Vascul Pharmacol.,* 2013; 58 (4):280-91.

[20] Schedin-Weiss S, Richard B, Hjelm R, Olson ST. Antiangiogenic forms of antithrombin specifically bind to the anticoagulant heparin sequence. *Biochemistry,* 2008; 47 (51):13610-9

[21] Pribluda VS, Gubish, Jr ER, LaVallee TM, Treston A, Swartz GM, Green SJ. 2-Methoxyestradiol: An endogenous antiangiogenic and antiproliferative drug candidate. *Cancer Metastasis Rev.,* 2000;19 (1-2):173 -9.

[22] Indraccolo S. Interferon-α as angiogenesis inhibitor: Learning from tumor models. *Autoimmunity,* 2010; 43 (3):244-7.

[23] Taylor KL, Leaman DW, Grane R, Mechti N, Borden EC, Lindner DJ. Identification of interferon-beta-stimulated genes that inhibit angiogenesis in vitro. *J. Interferon. Cytokine Res.,* 2008; 28 (12):733-40.

[24] Akhtar N1, Padilla ML, Dickerson EB, Steinberg H, Breen M, Auerbach R, et al. Interleukin-12 inhibits tumor growth in a novel angiogenesis canine hemangiosarcoma xenograft model. *Neoplasia,* 2004; 6 (2):106-16.

[25] Haas CS, Amin MA, Allen BB, Ruth JH, Haines GK 3rd, Woods JM, et al. Inhibition of Angiogenesis by Interleukin-4 Gene Therapy in Rat Adjuvant-Induced Arthritis. *Arthritis Rheum.,* 2006; 54 (8):2402-14.

[26] Subramanian P, Crawford SE, Becerra SP. Assays for the Antiangiogenic and Neurotrophic Serpin Pigment Epithelium-Derived Factor. *Methods Enzymol.,* 2011; 499:183–204.

[27] Paulus P, Jennewein C, Zacharowski K. Biomarkers of endothelial dysfunction: can they help us deciphering systemic inflammation and sepsis? *Biomarkers,* 2011; 16 (1):11–21.

[28] Vailhe B, Feige JJ. Thrombospondins as anti-angiogenic therapeutic agents. *Curr. Pharm. Des.,* 2003; 9 (7):583–8.

[29] Maharaj AS1, Walshe TE, Saint-Geniez M, Venkatesha S, Maldonado AE, Himes NC, Matharu KS, Karumanchi SA, D'Amore PA. *J. Exp. Med.,* 2008; 205:491-501.

[30] Sung HK1, Michael IP, Nagy A. Multifaceted role of vascular endothelial growth factor signaling in adult tissue physiology: an emerging concept with clinical implications. *Curr. Opin. Hematol.,* 2010; 17:206-12.

[31] Gibbons G. Endothelial function as a determinant of vascular function and structure: a new therapeutic target. *Am. J. Cardiol.,* 1997; 79 (5A): 3-8.

[32] van der Flier M, van Leeuwen HJ, van Kessel KP, Kimpen JL, Hoepelman AI, Geelen SP. Plasma vascular endothelial growth factor in severe sepsis. *Shock,* 2005; 23 (1):35-8.
[33] Liekens S, De Clercq E, Neyts J. Angiogenesis: regulators and clinical applications. *Biochem. Pharmacol.,* 2001; 61 (3):253-70
[34] Dehghanian F1, Hojati Z1, Kay M1. New Insights into VEGF-A Alternative Splicing: Key Regulatory Switching in the Pathological Process. *Avicenna J. Med. Biotechnol.,* 2014; 6:192-9.
[35] Thanigaimani S, Kichenadasse G, Mangoni AA. The emerging role of vascular endothelial growth factor (VEGF) in vascular homeostasis: lessons from recent trials with anti-VEGF drugs. *Curr. Vasc. Pharmacol.,* 2011; 9:358-80.
[36] Ferrara N, Davis-Smyth T. The biology of vascular endothelial growth factor. *Endocr. Rev.,* 1997; 18 (1): 4-25.
[37] Gerber H, Dixit V, Ferrara N. Vascular endothelial growth factor induces expression of the antiapoptotic proteins Bcl-2 and A1 in vascular endothelial cells. *J. Biol. Chem.,* 1998; 273 (21): 13313-6.
[38] Ashrafpour H, Huang N, Neligan PC, et al. Vasodilator effect and mechanism of action of vascular endothelial growth factor in skin vasculature. *Am. J. Physiol. Heart Circ. Physiol.,* 2004; 286 (3): 946-54.
[39] Abraham D, Hofbauer R, Schafer R, et al. Selective Downregulation of VEGF-A165, VEGF-R1, and decreased capillary density in patients with dilative but not ischemic cardiomyopathy. *Circ. Res.,* 2000; 87: 644.
[40] Roberts W, Palade G. Increased microvascular permeability and endothelial fenestration induced by vascular endothelial growth factor. *J. Cell Sci.,* 1995; 108 (Pt 6): 2369-79.
[41] Thomas M, Augustin HG. The role of the Angiopoietins in vascular morphogenesis. *Angiogenesis,* 2009;12 (2):125-37.
[42] Puri MC, Rossant J, Alitalo K, Bernstein A, Partanen J. The receptor tyrosine kinase TIE is required for integrity and survival of vascular endothelial cells. *EMBO J.,* 1995; 14 (23):5884–5891.
[43] Berse B, Hunt JA, Diegel RJ, Morganelli P, Yeo K, Brown F, et al. Hypoxia augments cytokine (transforming growth factor-beta (TGF-b) and IL-1)- induced vascular endothelial growth factor secretion by human synovial fibroblasts. *Clin. Exp. Immunol.,* 1999; 115 (1): 176-82.
[44] Fagiani E, Christofori G. Angiopoietins in angiogenesis. *Cancer Lett.,* 2013 1;328:18-26.
[45] Hammes HP, Lin J, Wagner P, Feng Y, Vom Hagen F, Krzizok T, et al. Angiopoietin-2 causes pericyte dropout in the normal retina: evidence

for involvement in diabetic retinopathy. *Diabetes,* 2004; 53 (4):1104–1110.

[46] Lobov IB, Brooks PC, Lang RA. Angiopoietin-2 displays VEGF-dependent modulation of capillary structure and endothelial cell survival in vivo. *Proc. Natl. Acad. Sci. USA,* 2002; 20;99 (17):11205-10

[47] Armulik A, Abramsson A, Betsholtz C. Endothelial/pericyte interactions. *Circ. Res.,* 2005; 97 (6):512–523.

[48] Ramsauer M, D'Amore PA. Contextual role for angiopoietins and TGFbeta1 in blood vessel stabilization. *J. Cell Sci.,* 2007; 120 (Pt 10):1810–1817.

[49] King EG, Bauzá GJ, Mella JR, Remick DG. Pathophysiologic mechanisms in septic shock. *Lab Invest.,* 2014; 94:4-12.

[50] Dellinger RP, Levy MM, Rhodes A, Annane D, Gerlach H, Opal SM, et al. Surviving Sepsis Campaign: International Guidelines for Management of Severe Sepsis and Septic Shock: 2012. *Intensive Care Med.,* 2013; 39:165-228

[51] De Backer D, Orbegozo Cortes D, Donadello K, Vincent JL. Pathophysiology of microcirculatory dysfunction and the pathogenesis of septic shock. *Virulence,* 2014; 5 (1):73-9.

[52] Remick DG. Pathophysiology of sepsis. *Am. J. Pathol.,* 2007; 170 (5):14 35-44.

[53] Macdonald J, Galley HF, Webster NR. Oxidative stress and gene expression in sepsis. *Br. J. Anaesth.,* 2003; 90 (2):221-32.

[54] Boisramé-Helms J, Kremer H, Schini-Kerth V, Meziani F. Endothelial dysfunction in sepsis. *Curr. Vasc. Pharmacol.,* 2013; 11 (2):150-60.

[55] Karapetsa M, Pitsika M, Goutzourelas N, Stagos D, Tousia Becker A, Zakynthinos E. Oxidative status in ICU patients with septic shock. *Food Chem. Toxicol., 2013*; 61:106-11.

[56] Valko M, Leibfritz D, Moncol J, Cronin MT, Mazur M, Telser J. Free radicals and antioxidants in normal physiological functions and human disease. *Int. J. Biochem. Cell Biol.,* 2007; 39 (1):44-84.

[57] Huet O, Dupic L, Harrois A, Duranteau J. Oxidative stress and endothelial dysfunction during sepsis. Front Biosci (Landmark Ed). 2011; 16:1986-95.

[58] Opal SM, van der Poll T. Endothelial barrier dysfunction in septic shock. *J. Intern. Med.,* 2014.

[59] Musa MG, Torrens C, Clough GF. The microvasculature: a target for nutritional programming and later risk of cardio-metabolic disease. *Acta Physiol.,* (Oxf). 2014; 210 (1):31-45.

[60] Gates PE, Strain WD, Shore AC. Human endothelial function and microvascular ageing. *Exp. Physiol.,* 2009; 94 (3):311-6.

[61] DeLano FA, Schmid-Schönbein GW, Skalak TC, Zweifach BW. Penetration of the systemic blood pressure into the microvasculature of rat skeletal muscle. *Microvasc. Res.,* 1991; 41 (1):92-110.

[62] Vallet B. Bench-to-bedside review: endothelial cell dysfunction in severe sepsis: a role in organ dysfunction? *Crit. Care,* 2003; 7 (2):130-8.

[63] Bateman RM, Tokunaga C, Kareco T, Dorscheid DR, Walley KR. Myocardial hypoxia-inducible HIF-1alpha, VEGF, and GLUT1 gene expression is associated with microvascular and ICAM-1 heterogeneity during endotoxemia. *Am. J. Physiol. Heart Circ Physiol.,* 2007; 293 (1): 448-56.

[64] Wester T, Häggblad E, Awan ZA, Barratt-Due A, Kvernebo M, Halvorsen PS, et al. Assessments of skin and tongue microcirculation reveals major changes in porcine sepsis. *Clin. Physiol. Funct Imaging,* 2011; 31 (2):151-8.

[65] De Backer D, Creteur J, Preiser JC, Dubois MJ, Vincent JL. Microvascular blood flow is altered in patients with sepsis. *Am. J. Respir. Crit. Care Med.,* 2002; 166 (1):98-104;

[66] Nencioni A, Trzeciak S, Shapiro NI. The microcirculation as a diagnostic and therapeutic target in sepsis. *Intern. Emerg. Med.,* 2009; 4 (5):413-8.

[67] Vincent JL, De Backer D. Microvascular dysfunction as a cause of organ dysfunction in severe sepsis. *Crit. Care,* 2005; 9 (4):9-12.

[68] Mittermayer F, Pleiner J, Schaller G, Weltermann A, Kapiotis S, Jilma B, et al. Marked increase in vascular endothelial growth factor concentrations during Escherichia coli endotoxin-induced acute inflammation in humans. *Eur. J. Clin. Invest.,* 2003; 33 (9):758-61.

[69] McCourt M, Wang JH, Sookhai S, Redmond HP. Proinflammatory mediators stimulate neutrophil-directed angiogenesis. *Arch. Surg.,* 1999; 134(12): 1325-31.

[70] Tsao PN, Chan FT, Wei SC, Hsieh WS, Chou HC, Su YN, et al. Soluble vascular endothelial growth factor receptor-1 protects mice in sepsis. *Crit. Care Med.,* 2007; 35 (8):1955-60.

[71] Kim I, Moon SO, Kim SH, Kim HJ, Koh YS, Koh GY. Vascular endothelial growth factor expression of intercellular adhesion molecule 1 (ICAM-1), vascular cell adhesion molecule 1 (VCAM-1), and E-selectin through nuclear factor-kappa B activation in endothelial cells. *J. Biol. Chem.,* 2001; 276 (10):7614-20.

[72] Kumpers P, van Meurs M, David S, Molema G, Bijzet J, Lukasz A, et al. Time course of angiopoietin-2 release during experimental human endotoxemia and sepsis. *Crit. Care,* 2009;13 (3):64.

[73] Fiedler U, Scharpfenecker M, Koidl S, Hegen A, Grunow V, Schmidt JM, et al. The Tie-2 ligand angiopoietin-2 is stored in and rapidly released upon stimulation from endothelial cell Weibel-Palade bodies. *Blood,* 2004;103 (11):4150-6.

[74] Hernandez G, Bruhn A, Ince C. Microcirculation in sepsis: new perspectives. *Curr. Vasc. Pharmacol.,* 2013; 11 (2):161-9.

[75] Sakr Y, Dubois MJ, De Backer D, Creteur J, Vincent JL. Persistent microcirculatory alterations are associated with organ failure and death in patients with septic shock. *Crit. Care Med.,* 2004; 32 (9):1825-31.

[76] van Zanten AR, Brinkman S, Arbous MS, Abu-Hanna A, Levy MM, de Keizer NF, Netherlands Patient Safety Agency Sepsis Expert Group. Guideline bundles adherence and mortality in severe sepsis and septic shock. *Crit. Care Med.,* 2014; 42 (8):1890-8.

[77] Levy MM, Rhodes A, Phillips GS, Townsend SR, Schorr CA, Beale R, et al. Surviving Sepsis Campaign: association between performance metrics and outcomes in a 7.5-year study. *Intensive Care Med.,* 2014; 40:1623-33.

[78] Ferrer R, Martin-Loeches I, Phillips G, Osborn TM, Townsend S, Dellinger RP, et al. Empiric antibiotic treatment reduces mortality in severe sepsis and septic shock from the first hour: results from a guideline-based performance improvement program. *Crit. Care Med.,* 2014; 42 (8):1749-55.

[79] Shapiro NI, Arnold R, Sherwin R, O'Connor J, Najarro G, Singh S, et al. The association of near-infrared spectroscopy-derived tissue oxygenation measurements with sepsis syndromes, organ dysfunction and mortality in emergency department patients with sepsis. *Crit. Care,* 2011;15 (5):223.

[80] De Backer D, Donadello K, Sakr Y, Ospina-Tascon G, Salgado D, Scolletta S, et al. Microcirculatory alterations in patients with severe sepsis: impact of time of assessment and relationship with outcome. *Crit. Care Med.,* 2013; 41 (3):791-9.

[81] Sharawy N. Vasoplegia in septic shock: do we really fight the right enemy? *J. Crit. Care,* 2014; 29 (1):83-7

[82] Umans JG, Wylam ME, Samsel RW, Edwards J, Schumacker PT. Effects of endotoxin in vivo on endothelial and smooth-muscle function

in rabbit and rat aorta. *Am. Rev. Respir. Dis.,* 1993; 148 (6 Pt 1):1638-45.

[83] Levy B, Collin S, Sennoun N, Ducrocq N, Kimmoun A, Asfar P, et al. Vascular hyporesponsiveness to vasopressors in septic shock: from bench to bedside. *Intensive Care Med.,* 2010; 36 (12):2019-29.

[84] Wu CC, Szabó C, Chen SJ, Thiemermann C, Vane JR. Activation of soluble guanylyl cyclase by a factor other than nitric oxide or carbon monoxide contributes to the vascular hyporeactivity to vasoconstrictor agents in the aorta of rats treated with endotoxin. *Biochem. Biophys. Res. Commun.,* 1994; 201(1):436-42.

[85] Underbakke ES, Iavarone AT, Chalmers MJ, Pascal BD, Novick S, Griffin PR, et al. Nitric oxide-induced conformational changes in soluble guanylate cyclase. *Structure,* 2014; 22 (4):602-11.

[86] Hecker M, Cattaruzza M, Wagner AH. Regulation of inducible nitric oxide synthase gene expression in vascular smooth muscle cells. *Gen Pharmacol.,* 1999; 32 (1):9-16.

[87] Cauwels A. Nitric oxide in shock. *Kidney Int.,* 2007; 72 (5):557 65

[88] Endemann DH, Schiffrin EL. Endothelial dysfunction. *J. Am. Soc. Nephrol.,* 2004; 15 (8):1983-92.

[89] He H, Venema VJ, Gu X, Venema RC, Marrero MB, Caldwell RB. Vascular endothelial growth factor signals endothelial cell production of nitric oxide and prostacyclin through flk-1/KDR activation of c-Src. *J. Biol. Chem.,* 1999; 274 (35): 25130–25135.

[90] Goldenberg NM, Steinberg BE, Slutsky AS, Lee WL. Broken barriers: a new take on sepsis pathogenesis. *Sci. Transl. Med.,* 2011; 3(88):88ps25.

[91] London NR, Zhu W, Bozza FA, et al. Targeting Robo4-dependent Slit signaling to survive the cytokine storm in sepsis and influenza. *Sci. Transl. Med.,* 2010; 2(23):23ra19.

[92] Henrich M, Gruss M, Weigand MA. Sepsis-induced degradation of endothelial glycocalyx. *Scientific World Journal,* 2010; 10:917-23.

[93] Alphonsus CS1, Rodseth RN. The endothelial glycocalyx: a review of the vascular barrier. *Anaesthesia,* 2014; 69:777-84.

[94] Witzenbichler B, Westermann D, Knueppel S, Schultheiss HP, Tschope C. Protective role of angiopoietin-1 in endotoxic shock. *Circulation,* 2005; 111 (1):97-105.

[95] Parikh SM, Mammoto T, Schultz A, Yuan HT, Christiani D, Karumanchi SA, et al. Excess circulating angiopoietin-2 may contribute to pulmonary vascular leak in sepsis in humans. *PLoS Med.,* 2006; 3(3):46.

[96] Mammoto T, Parikh SM, Mammoto A, Gallagher D, Chan B, Mostoslavsky G, et al. Angiopoietin-1 requires p190 RhoGAP to protect against vascular leakage in vivo. *J. Biol. Chem.,* 2007; 282 (33):23910-8.

[97] Salmon AH, Neal CR, Sage LM, Glass CA, Harper SJ, Bates DO. Angiopoietin-1 alters microvascular permeability coefficients in vivo via modification of endothelial glycocalyx. *Cardiovasc. Res.,* 2009; 83(1): 24-33.

[98] Dvorak HF, Brown LF, Detmar M, Dvorak AM. Vascular permeability factor/vascular endothelial growth factor, microvascular hyperper meability, and angiogenesis. Am J Pathol 1995; 146 (5):1029–1039.

[99] Pocock TM, Williams B, Curry FE, Bates DO. VEGF and ATP act by different mechanisms to increase microvascular permeability and endothelial [Ca(2+)]. *Am. J. Physiol. Heart Circ. Physiol.,* 2000; 279 (4):1625-34.

[100] Tiruppathi C1, Ahmmed GU, Vogel SM, Malik AB. Ca2+ signaling, TRP channels, and endothelial permeability. *Microcirculation,* 2006; 13 (8):693-708.

[101] León C, Loza A. Biomarcadores en la sepsis. ¿Simplicando lo complejo? Enferm Infecc *Microbiol. Clin.,* 2014;32(3):137–139.

[102] Biomakers Definitions Working Group. Biomarkers and surrogate endpoints: Preferred definitions and conceptual framework. *Clin. Pharmacol. Ther.,* 2011; 69 (3): 89-95.

[103] Pierrakos C, Vincent JL. Sepsis biomarkers: a review. *Crit. Care,* 2010; 14(1):R15.

[104] Zhang R-Y, Liu Y-Y, Qu H-P, Tang Y-Q. The angiogenic factors and their soluble receptors in sepsis: friend, foe, or both? *Crit. Care,* 2013; 17 (4):446.

[105] Karlsson S, Pettila V, Tenhunen J, Lund V, Hovilehto S, Ruokonen E. Vascular Endothelial Growth Factor in Severe Sepsis and Septic Shock. *Anesth Analg.,* 2008; 106 (6): 1820-6.

[106] Jesmin S, Wada T, Gando S, Sultana SS, Zaedi S. The Dynamics of Angiogenic Factors and Their Soluble Receptors in Relation to Organ Dysfunction in Disseminated Intravascular Coagulation Associated with Sepsis. *Inflammation,* 2013; 36(1): 186-96.

[107] Liu Y, Song S-D, Wang H-X. [A clinical study of the serum vascular endothelial growth factor in patients with severe sepsis]. Zhongguo Wei Zhong Bing Ji Jiu Yi Xue. 2009; 21 (3): 172-174.

[108] Ostrowski S, Sørensen AM, Windeløv NA, Perner A, Welling K-L, Wanscher M, et al. High levels of soluble VEGF receptor 1 early after

trauma are associated with shock, sympathoadrenal activation, glycocalyx degradation and inflammation in severely injured patients: a prospective study. *Sc. and J. Trauma Resusc Emerg Med.,* 2012; 20: 27.

[109] Schuetz P, Jones AE, Aird WC, Shapiro NI. Endothelial Cell Activation in Emergency Department Patients with Sepsis and Non-Sepsis related Hypotension. *Shock,* 2011; 36 (2): 104-108.

[110] Alves BE, Montalvao SA, Aranha FJP, Lorand-Metze I, De Souza CA, Annichino-Bizzacchi JM, et al. Time course of sFlt-1 and VEGF-A release in neutropenic patients with sepsis and septic shock: a prospective study. *J. Transl. Med.,* 2011; 9:23.

[111] Yang K-Y, Liu K-T, Chen Y-C, Chen C-S, Lee Y-C, Perng R-P, Feng J-Y. Plasma soluble vascular endothelial growth factor receptor-1 levels predict outcomes of pneumonia-related septic shock patients: a prospective observational study. *Crit. Care,* 2011; 15(1):R11.

[112] Skibsted S, Jones AE, Puskarich MA, Arnold R, Sherwin R, Trzeciak S, et al. Biomarkers of endothelial cell activation in early sepsis. *Shock,* 2013; 39(5): 427-432.

[113] Page AV, Liles WC. Biomarkers of endothelial activation/dysfunction in infectious diseases. *Virulence,* 2013; 4 (6): 507-516.

[114] Cho S-Y, Choi J-H. Biomarkers of Sepsis. *Infect. Chemother.,* 2014; 46 (1): 1-12.

[115] Davis JS, Weo TW, Piera KA, Woodberry T, Celermajer DS, Stephens DP, et al. Angiopoietin-2 is increased in sepsis and inversely associated with nitric oxide-dependent microvascular reactivity. *Crit. Care,* 2010; 14(3):R89.

[116] Giuliano JS Jr, Wheeler DS. Excess circulating angiopoietin-2 levels in sepsis: harbinger of death in the intensive care unit? *Crit. Care,* 2009; 13 (1):114.

[117] Orfanos SE, Kotanidou A, Glynos C, Athanasiou C, Tsigkos S, Dimopolou I, et al. Angiopoietin-2 is increased in severe sepsis: correlation with inflammatory mediators. *Crit. Care Med.,* 2007; 35 (1): 199 206.

[118] Wada T, Jesmin S, Gando S, Yanagida Y, Mizugaki A, Sultana S, et al. The role of angiogenic factors and their soluble receptors in acute lung injury (ALI)/ acute respiratory distress syndrome (ARDS) associated with critical illness. *J. Inflamm.,* (Lond). 2013; 10(1):6.

[119] David S, van Meurs M, Kümpers P. Does low angiopoietin-1 predict adverse outcome in sepsis? *Crit. Care,* 2010; 14(4):180.

[120] Ricciuto DR, Dos Santos CC, Hawkes M, Toltl LJ, Conroy AL, Rajwans N, et al. Angiopoietin-1 and angiopoietin-2 as clinically informative prognostic biomarkers of morbidity and mortality in severe sepsis. *Crit. Care Med.,* 2011. 39 (4): 702-710.

[121] Walley KR. Biomarkers in Sepsis. *Curr. Infect. Dis. Rep.,* 2013; 15:413–420

[122] Xing K, Murthy S, Liles WC, Singh JM. Clinical utility of biomarkers of endothelial activation in sepsis- a systematic review. *Crit. Care,* 2012; 16(1):R7.

[123] Jeong SJ, Han SH, Kim CO, Choi JY, Kim JM. Anti-vascular endothelial growth factor antibody attenuates inflammation and decreases mortality in an experimental model of severe sepsis. *Crit. Care,* 2013;17(3):R97.

[124] Ferrara N, Gerber HP, LeCouter J. The biology of VEGF and its receptors. *Nat. Med.,* 2003; 9(6):669 – 76.

[125] Kumpers P, Gueler F, David S, Slyke PV, Dumont DJ, Park JK, Bockmeyer CL, Parikh SM, Pavenstadt H, Haller H, Shushakova N. The synthetic tie2 agonist peptide vasculotide protects against vascular leakage and reduces mortality in murine abdominal sepsis. *Crit. Care,* 2011;15(5):261.

[126] David S, Park JK, Meurs Mv, Zijlstra JG, Koenecke C, Schrimpf C, et al. Acute administration of recombinant Angiopoietin-1 ameliorates multiple-organ dysfunction syndrome and improves survival in murine sepsis. *Cytokine,* 2011; 55(2):251-9.

[127] Ziegler T, Horstkotte J, Schwab C, Pfetsch V, Weinmann K, Dietzel S, et al. Angiopoietin 2 mediates microvascular and hemodynamic alterations in sepsis. *J. Clin. Invest.,* 2013;123(8): 3436–4.

In: Septic Shock
Editor: Benedict Graver

ISBN: 978-1-63463-916-3

Chapter IV

Membrane-Bound and Soluble Triggered Receptor Expressed on Myeloid Cells 1 (TREM-1) Discriminates Sepsis from Other Causes of Systemic Inflammation

Ioannis Gkougkourellas**, *Alexandros Sarantopoulos, Konstantinos Tselios, Athanasios Kalogeridis, Marianna Pantoura, Anastasia Georgiadou, Spyros Gerou and Panagiota Boura

Clinical Immunology Unit, 2nd Department of Internal Medicine,
Hippokration General Hospital,
Aristotle University of Thessaloniki, Greece

* Corresponding Author: Ioannis Gkougkourellas, Clinical Immunology Unit, 2nd Department of Internal Medicine, Hippokration General Hospital, Aristotle University of Thessaloniki, Konstantinoupoleos St. 49, 546 42, Thessaloniki, Greece, Tel: 00302-310-892239, Fax: 00302-310-992794, E-mail: igkougkourelas@gmail.com

Abstract

Background and Objective: Accurate differential diagnosis between sepsis and other, non-infectious, causes of systemic inflammatory response syndrome (SIRS) is crucial for timely intervention and survival; however, no single biomarker can confirm pathogen presence in such patients. In this context, we assessed Triggered Receptor Expressed on Myelocytes-1 (TREM-1, soluble and membrane-bound forms), a molecule known to propagate systemic inflammation, in regard to its diagnostic value.

Patients and Methods: Seventy patients were enrolled in total. Group A consisted of 37 adult patients with sepsis, mean age 69.7±15.2 years, diagnosed according to the 2011 Sepsis International Conference criteria (10 with severe sepsis/septic shock and 27 without any organ damage). Group B included 16 patients with systemic autoimmune inflammation (non-infectious SIRS), 8 of them with active rheumatoid arthritis (RA, mean age 65±21 years, Disease Activity Score=4.8±0.8) and 8 with active systemic lupus erythematosus (SLE, mean age 45±5 years, SLE Disease Activity Index=8±2). Group C consisted of 17 healthy individuals for establishing a reference point. Traditional biomarkers, such as C-reactive protein (CRP) and procalcitonin (PCT) were available in the majority of patients. TREM-1 expression on CD14+ monocytes was assessed with flow-cytometry whereas soluble TREM-1 was measured with enzyme-linked immunosorbent assay (ELISA). Statistical analysis was performed with Mann-Whitney U test; $p<0.05$ was considered significant.

Results: TREM-1 expression on CD14+ macrophages was significantly enhanced in septic patients (50.19±15.79%) in comparison to autoimmune patients (28.2±14%, $p<0.05$) and healthy controls (16.2±10%, $p<0.05$). Likewise, soluble TREM-1 levels were significantly higher in group A (124.6±36.1pg/ml) than group B (43.6±17.4pg/ml, $p<0.05$) and healthy individuals (5±3.3pg/ml, $p<0.05$). Of note, both membrane-bound and soluble TREM-1 did not differ significantly between patients with severe sepsis/septic shock and those without any overt organ damage.

Conclusion: Patients with sepsis and severe sepsis/septic shock have significantly higher levels of the membrane-bound and soluble forms of TREM-1 compared to active autoimmune patients and healthy individuals. TREM-1 may accurately discriminate infectious from non-infectious SIRS causes.

Keywords: Sepsis, biomarker, triggered receptor expressed on myeloid cells-1

Introduction

Sepsis is among the most common causes of death in hospitalized patients; its incidence is increasing approximately 8.7%/year, resulting in 240.4 cases per 100000 inhabitants in 2000, probably due to the aging of population and the increased use of immunosuppressive medications or chemotherapy. [1] Although considerable progress in the management of critically ill patients has been achieved, sepsis remains an ominous diagnosis. In-hospital mortality ranges from 28.3 to 41.1% in North America and Europe. [1, 2] One third of the septic patients will die from direct complications, such as remote organ dysfunction (severe sepsis) and/or arterial hypotension (septic shock). Many patients may deteriorate unrecognized, as occurrence of infection and related organ dysfunction eludes from physician' s attention. The high rates of delayed diagnosis are frustrating, since it is well documented that every hour of delay in management of sepsis may increase mortality by 10%. [3]

Up-to date sepsis diagnosis relies on the identification of Systemic Inflammatory Response Syndrome (SIRS) and a severe, uncontrolled infection. SIRS criteria are a) tachycardia >90/min, b) tachypnea >20 breaths/min or $PaCO_2$ <32 mmHg c) fever (>38°C) or hypothermia (<36°C) and d) altered white blood cell count (WBC>12,000 cells/mm^3 or <4000 cells/mm^3) or presence of >10% immature neutrophils on peripheral blood smear. Sepsis is defined as SIRS resulting from infection, whether of bacterial, viral, fungal or parasitic origin. Diagnosis is reached when 2 or more of the above conditions are met. [4]

SIRS criteria are characterized by a high sensitivity but low specificity, thus resulting in relatively poor diagnostic accuracy. [5] Besides overwhelming infections, other causes of SIRS include trauma, acute pancreatitis, burns and, rarely, autoimmune diseases such as systemic lupus erythematosus (SLE) and highly active rheumatoid arthritis (RA). [6] In typical cases, severe infections are well differentiated from aseptic patients with signs of SIRS, however, sometimes, differential diagnosis is challenging. Traditional markers of systemic inflammation, such as WBC, erythrocyte sedimentation rate (ESR) and C-reactive protein (CRP) have been proven of limited value in such patients due to their poor sensitivity and specificity for infection. [7] Moreover, microbiological (bodily fluid and tissue) cultures, the conventional gold standard for sepsis diagnosis, are time consuming and, thus, unsuitable for early diagnosis. Additionally, any widely available laboratory investigation cannot precisely determine the host response in cases of SIRS/sepsis or the exact onset of organ dysfunction whereas, sometimes, is misleading with false-positive or false-negative results. [8] Given this evidence, differential diagnosis of sepsis from other causes of SIRS has become a hot topic in late years. [9] These shortcomings in both clinical and laboratory tests have driven researchers to find other, more sensitive and specific markers.

Though CRP and procalcitonin (PCT) are currently used as biochemical indicators of inflammation and infection, several other biomarkers have been investigated for their ability to detect sepsis in an early, reversible stage. [10] Diagnostic accuracy of PCT has been investigated in meta-analyses, showing a modest capability to discriminate sepsis, since the estimated likelihood ratio of PCT was approximately 7.5, value of modest performance. [11]

Nonetheless, identification of an ideal biomarker (or panel of biomarkers), capable of making a clear distinction between sepsis and SIRS, is imperative. [10] Several biomarkers such as interleukins, pro-vasopressin, CD64 etc. have been tested for the diagnosis, assessment and prognosis of sepsis. Except for PCT, however, their clinical value is still uncertain or controversial. [9, 10. 12, 13, 14]

In 2004, triggering receptor expressing on myeloid cells-1 (TREM-1) was evaluated for its accuracy in the diagnosis and evaluation of sepsis by Gibot et al. [15] TREM-1 is involved in the activation of innate immunity cells and the inflammatory response. It belongs to the immunoglobulin superfamily, engaged as a cell membrane receptor; mainly in the family of myeloid cells. [16] Its expression on monocytes and neutrophils is altered when a pattern recognition receptor (PRR), such as Toll-like receptor (TLR)-4, is activated by a pathogen-associated molecular pattern (PAMP). In vitro activation of TREM-1, in the presence of TLR-2 or TLR-4 ligands, amplifies the production of proinflammatory cytokines, such as tumour necrosis factor (TNF-α), IL-1β and granulocyte–macrophage colony-stimulating factor (GM-CSF). Simultaneously, it inhibits the release of the regulatory cytokine IL-10, further promoting the inflammatory response. [16, 17] The ligand of TREM-1 has not been identified yet. Its action is mediated through the DAP12 protein, whereas other studies have shown that TREM-1 is activated through a phosphatidylinositol-3-kinase-dependent (PI3K) pathway. In parallel, when TLRs are stimulated, the production of the soluble form of TREM-1 (sTREM-1) is augmented. [18] sTREM-1 could originate from the shedding of the membrane bound receptor (mTREM-1) by a metalloprotease or an alternative splicing of the mRNA.[16] Soluble TREM-1 acts as a decoy receptor, sequestering TREM-1 ligand and dampening its activation. Moreover, up-regulation of mTREM-1 may result in marked elevation of the soluble form in plasma. [12]

In mice, engagement of TREM-1 with monoclonal agonist antibodies was shown to stimulate the production of pro-inflammatory cytokines and chemokines, such as IL-8, monocyte chemoattractant protein-1 (MCP)-1 and -3, and macrophage inflammatory protein-1 (MIP-1), leading to rapid neutrophil degranulation and oxidative burst. [17] Pro-inflammatory cytokine secretion (IL-8, IL-6 and TNF-α) was significantly compromised when leukocytes were treated with the synthetic peptide LP17, which may act as a decoy receptor, by blocking interaction of TREM-1 with its ligand. The inflammatory response mediated by TLR-2 and TLR-4 stimulation is amplified by the engagement of mTREM-1. [18] Modulation of TREM-1 signaling pathway, with the use of small synthetic peptides, confers considerable survival advantages during experimental septic shock in mice, even if they are administered late after the onset of sepsis. [19, 20]

mTREM-1 expression on circulating CD14+ monocytes and tissue macrophages is up-regulated, when infection by Gram-positive and Gram-negative bacteria occurs. During sepsis, in particular, the expression of mTREM-1 is greatly increased on monocytes, albeit reduced on neutrophils. [21]

Gibot et al. investigated whether sepsis alters mTREM-1 expression, using experimental models of polymicrobial infection induced by caecal ligation and puncture (CLP) in mice. In sham-operated animals, TREM-1 was present at low levels on the surface of peripheral monocytes and neutrophils, peritoneal macrophages and neutrophils, as well as splenic macrophages. Sepsis induced a marked (three-fold to five-fold) increase in TREM-1 expression on the surface of CD14+ cells, with the most pronounced increase observed on peritoneal macrophages. Furthermore, the release of sTREM-1 was substantially increased in peritoneal lavage fluid from septic animals but it was barely detectable in sham-operated animals. [22] Other studies have shown that its expression is dramatically increased in skin, biological fluids and tissues infected by Gram-positive and Gram-negative bacteria and fungi. [23, 24] Additionally, elevated broncho-alveolar lavage fluid sTREM-1 concentrations were found in patients with bacterial or fungal pneumonia and increased pleural fluid sTREM-1 levels were detected in patients with infectious pleural effusions. [25]

Gibot and Cravoisy found that sTREM-1 displayed greater diagnostic value when compared to CRP and PCT and could represent a useful biomarker for early diagnosis of sepsis. [26] Other investigators found that TREM-1 increase may positively correlate to the critical condition and prognosis of the patients. [27]

Accordingly, other studies have shown that TREM-1 is not elevated in the serum of patients with non-infectious inflammatory disorders such as ulcerative colitis or immune-complex vasculitis, proposing TREM-1 as the ideal biomarker for the discrimination between septic and aseptic causes of SIRS. [12, 16, 28] On the contrary, reports that increased plasma sTREM-1 concentrations were also observed in patients with acute pancreatitis and non-infectious inflammations after traumatic lung contusion or pulmonary aspiration syndromes have been published. [29] Prucha et al. compared levels of mTREM-1 (assessed by flow cytometry) in septic patients and patients after CNS elective surgery and came to the conclusion that TREM-1 was increased in both entities. [30] The diagnostic and prognostic performance of sTREM-1 in sepsis and septic shock was reported to be variable and controversial, according to other clinical studies that reaffirmed the role of traditional laboratory parameters, such as CRP, IL-6 and PCT, in distinguishing sepsis from non-infectious SIRS. [31, 32] Latour-Pérez et al. assessed the accuracy of sTREM-1 and concluded that the area under the curve (AUC) of sTREM-1 for the diagnosis of sepsis was 0.62 [95% confidence interval (CI) 0.51-0.72]. Furthermore, the alterations of sTREM-1 had a modest diagnostic accuracy in the first three days after admission (P=0.047, sensitivity=47%, specificity=78%). [33]

In 2012, Gibot et al. introduced the concept of Bioscore (BS), which is a composite index, based on the measurement of three different biomarkers: sTREM-1, PCT and CD64. The authors assessed the ability of BS to achieve greater diagnostic accuracy in early sepsis. Three hundred intensive care unit (ICU) patients were studied and levels of these biomarkers were determined in 2 different blood samples that were obtained at 12 and 24 hours after admission. They defined a lower threshold (cut-off) for each biomarker (PCT: 1.55 ng/ml, sTREM-1: 755 pg/ml, PMNCD64 index: 1.62). Scoring of all parameters above the respective threshold in a combined BS confers a considerable diagnostic accuracy (AUC 0.97). [34] Moreover, a recent systematic review and meta-analysis evaluated the accuracy of plasma sTREM-1 for sepsis diagnosis in systemic inflammatory patients. The positive likelihood ratio, negative likelihood ratio and diagnostic odds ratio were 4.0 (95% CI, 2.4 to 6.9), 0.26 (95% CI, 0.14 to 0.48) and 16 (95% CI, 5 to 46) respectively. [35]

Given these discrepancies, aim of the present study was to compare the levels of TREM-1 expression on CD14+ cells and in serum in three groups of subjects: in patients with sepsis, in patients with autoimmune systemic inflammation and in healthy controls, in order to evaluate the diagnostic accuracy of TREM-1 in the discrimination between infectious and non-infectious causes of SIRS.

Patients and Methods

Seventy individuals were enrolled and subdivided as follows. Group A consisted of 37 adult patients (mean age 69.7±15.2 years) with sepsis, diagnosed according to the 2012 Sepsis International Conference criteria. [4] Septic patients were recruited between February 2010 and August 2012 from the Emergency Department (11 patients), the 2nd Department of Internal Medicine and the ICU of Hippokration General Hospital (26 patients). Exclusion criteria were age <14 years, pregnancy and use of immunosuppressive agents. The most frequent diagnosis, at the time of admission, was community acquired pneumonia (CAP) in 32% (n=12) of patients, followed by urinary tract infection in 25% (n=9), skin and soft tissue infection in 16% (n=6), catheter-related infection in 16% (n=6) and infection of unknown origin in 11% (n=4). Ten of these patients were suffering from severe sepsis/septic shock (subgroup A1) and 27 did not have any sign of end organ damage at the time of diagnosis (subgroup A2). Subdivision was made in accordance with the criteria of the American College of Chest Physicians/Society of Critical Care Medicine Consensus Conference for sepsis and severe sepsis/septic shock. [4]

Severe sepsis group was defined by the sepsis patients with more than one of organ dysfunction signs including (1) cardiovascular: arterial systolic blood pressure less than 90mmHg or mean arterial pressure less than 70mmHg that responds to administration of intravenous fluid, (2) renal: urine output less than 0.5mL/kg/hour for 1 hour despite adequate fluid resuscitation, (3) respiratory: PaO_2/FiO_2 less than 250, (4) hematologic: platelet count less than 80000/μL or 50% decrease in platelet count from highest value recorded over the previous 3 days, (5) unexplained metabolic acidosis: pH<7.30 or a base deficit>5.0 mEq/L and a plasma lactate level more than 1.5 times the upper limit of normal for reporting laboratory, (6) pulmonary artery wedge pressure less than 12 mmHg or central venous pressure less than 8 mmHg with adequate fluid resuscitation and (7) acute alteration of mental status. Septic shock was defined as sepsis with hypotension (systolic blood pressure below 90 mmHg or its reduction by 40 mmHg or more from baseline in the absence of other causes) despite adequate fluid resuscitation along with organ dysfunction signs or need of inotropes or vasopressors for maintaining a systolic blood pressure of more than 90 mmHg or mean arterial pressure of more than 70 mmHg. Laboratory tests such as CRP, PCT and blood, sputum and urine cultures were performed as a routine. The percentage of patients with positive blood cultures was 70%.

Table 1. Demographic characteristics, SIRS criteria and types of infections in our patients

Parameter	Group A (n=37)	Group B (n=16)
Age (years, mean±SD)	69.7±15.2	55±11
Female/male ratio	20/17	14/2
SIRS criteria		
Fever	35/37 (94%)	8/16 (50%)
Tachycardia	30/37 (81%)	12/16 (75%)
Tachypnea	10/37 (27%)	1/16 (6%)
White blood cells disturbances	30/37 (81%)	12/16 (75%)
Infection characteristics		
Septic shock	10/37 (27%)	
Community acquired pneumonia (CAP)	12/37 (32%)	
Skin and soft tissue infection	6/37 (16%)	
Urinary tract infection	9/37 (25%)	
Catheter-related infection	6/37 (16%)	
Infection of unknown origin	4/37 (11%)	

Group B included 16 patients with systemic autoimmune inflammation (non-infectious SIRS), 8 of them with active RA (mean age 65±21 years, Disease Activity Score=4.8±0.8) and 8 with active SLE (mean age 45±5 years, SLE Disease Activity Index=8±2). These patients were recruited from the Clinical Immunology Outpatient Clinic of the 2nd Department Internal Medicine and were newly diagnosed, without taking immunosuppressive medications. All RA patients had destructive arthritis and extra-articular manifestations as well (3 had rheumatoid nodules, 3 had rheumatoid lung and 2 had serositis). SLE patients had fever, hematologic abnormalities and visceral disease (2 with neurological manifestations, 3 with nephritis, and 3 with serositis). Diagnosis was made according to EULAR and ACR revised criteria respectively. [36, 37] SIRS criteria were satisfied in all patients.

Group C consisted of 17 healthy individuals (mean age 55±30 years) for establishing a reference point. Health status was confirmed by clinical examination and routine laboratory tests. Patients' characteristics are shown in Table 1.

Laboratory Methods

Flow Cytometry

Immunophenotypic analysis was performed on peripheral blood using three colour flow cytometry (EPICS COULTER XL®). Monoclonal antibodies used were: FITC-labeled anti-TLR4 (Clone 610015, R&D Systems®, Minneapolis, USA), PE-labeled anti-TREM-1 (Clone 193015, R&D Systems®, Minneapolis, USA) and PC5-labeled anti-CD14 (Clone RMO52, Beckman-Coulter®, Switzerland). Whole blood was incubated with the antibodies at 18°C for 15 minutes in the dark. Lysing and WBC membrane stabilization was performed by treatment of the specimen with prepared solutions (Immunoprep Reagent System, Beckman-Coulter®). A minimum of 2,000 cells was analyzed in each sample. Stained IgG_1 FITC and PE monoclonal antibodies mixed with CD14 PC5 antibody were used to determine negative control fluorescence for TLR4 and TREM-1 on macrophages.

Enzyme Linked Immunosorbent Assay (ELISA)

Levels of sTREM-1 in peripheral whole blood were measured by commercially available specific ELISA kits (USCN Life Sciences®) following the manufacturer's protocol. Each 100μl serum sample was transferred to the microstrip wells of the ELISA plate and subsequently incubated for 2 hour at 37°C; then the first reagent was added. After this, the plate was again incubated for 1 hour at 37°C. After 3 washing steps, the detection antibody was added and the reaction system was incubated for 30 min at 37°C. Antibody binding was detected using streptavidin-conjugated horseradish peroxidase and developed using a substrate solution. The reaction was then stopped by the addition of sulphoric acid solution and the optical density was determined spectrometrically using a microplate reader set at 450±10nm with a wavelength correction set at 570 nm to subtract background. Soluble TREM-1 concentration was measured according to a calibration curve using a human sTREM-1 standard. According to manufacturer's instructions, a standard curve was generated using a four-parameter logistic curve fit for each set of samples assayed. The lower limit detection of the test was 3.8 pg/ml. All the values were within the linear portion of the standard curve. The inter- and intra-assay coefficient of variation for the sTREM-1 tests were <10%.

Statistical Analysis

Results are expressed as mean±SD. Kruskal-Wallis test for independent variables was applied for differences' identification between the three groups.

The Mann-Whitney U-test was performed to assess the significant differences; $p<0.05$ was considered statistically significant. Spearman test was used for correlation assessment. All analyses were performed using the SigmaStat 4.0 software.

Results

TREM-1 expression on CD14+ macrophages (mTREM-1) was significantly enhanced in septic patients (mean value 50.19±15.79%) in comparison to autoimmune patients (mean value 28.2±14%, $p<0.05$) and healthy controls (mean value 16.2±10%, $p<0.05$), Table 2 and Figure 1. Likewise, soluble TREM-1 (sTREM-1) levels were significantly higher in group A (124.6±36.1 pg/ml) than group B (43.6±17.4 pg/ml, $p<0.05$) and healthy individuals (5±3.3 pg/ml, $p<0.05$), Table 2 and Figure 2).

Table 2. Expression of membrane TREM-1 on CD14+ monocytes of the peripheral blood and soluble receptor concentration in serum in the three groups

	Group A	Group B	Group C
Membrane TREM-1 on CD14+ cells (%)	50.19±15.79	28.2±14	16.2±10
sTREM-1 (pg/ml)	124.6±36.1	43.6±17.4	5±3.3

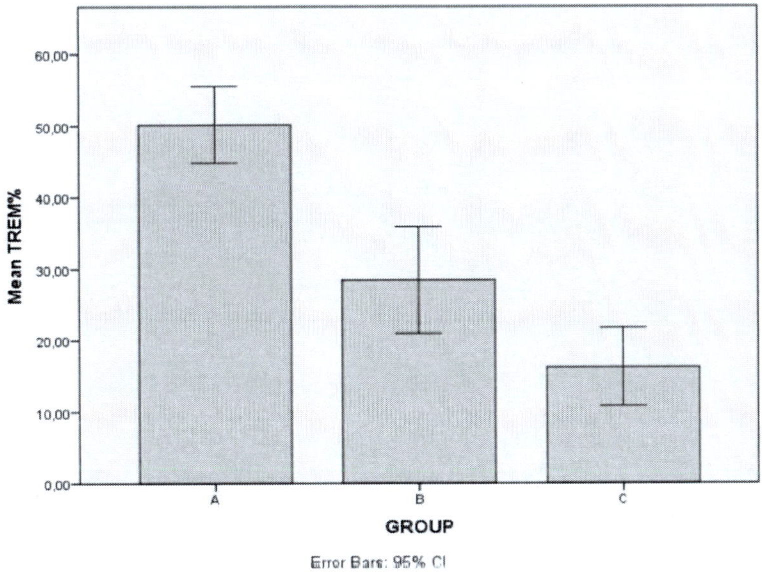

Figure 1. Cellular expression of membrane TREM-1 in the three groups.

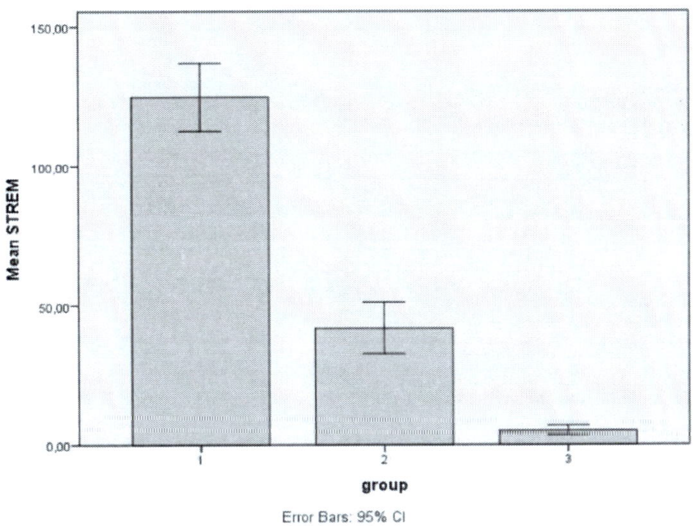

Figure 2. Serum concentrations of TREM-1 in the three groups.

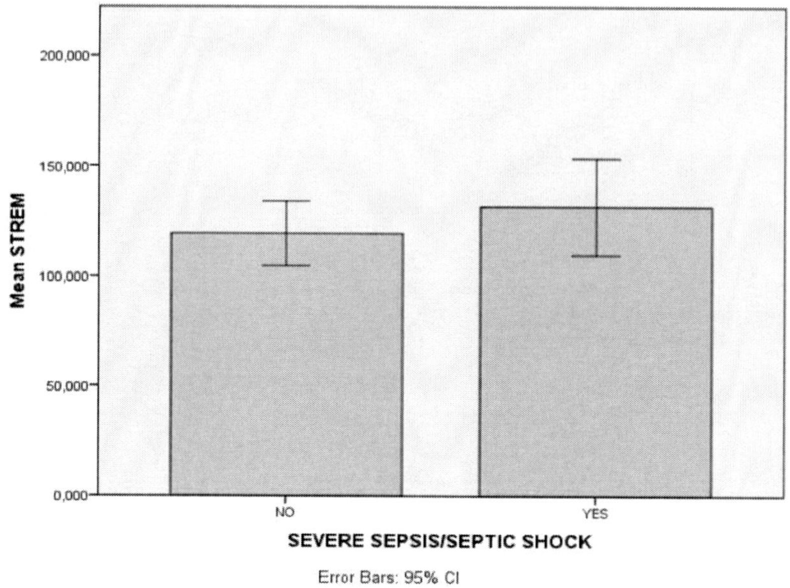

Figure 3. No statistical difference in sTREM-1 concentrations between subgroups A1 and A2.

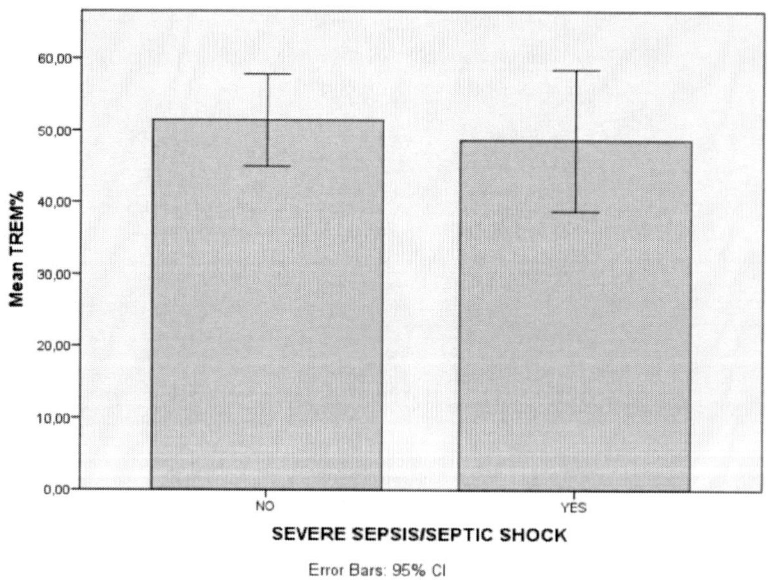

Figure 4. No statistical difference in mTREM% between subgroups A1 and A2.

The levels of sTREM-1 in healthy subjects were almost undetectable whereas the estimated expression of the membrane bound receptor was considered to be the basal expression in health.

Of note, both membrane-bound and soluble TREM-1 did not differ significantly between patients with severe sepsis/septic shock and those without any overt organ damage. The mean value of sTREM-1 in group A1 was 110±18 pg/ml whereas for group A2 was 125±28 pg/ml ($p>0.05$), Figure 3. Membrane bound receptor expression was 52.2±14% for group A1 and 48±10.79% for group A2, Figure 4 and Table 3.

TREM-1 on monocytes did correlate with serum TREM-1 in patients without severe sepsis ($r=0.54$, $p<0.05$) but not in uncomplicated sepsis ($r=0.33$, $p>0.05$), data not shown.

Table 3. Expression of membrane TREM-1 on peripheral blood CD14+ monocytes and soluble receptor concentration in serum in subgroups A1 and A2

	Group A1	Group A2
Membrane TREM-1 on CD14+ cells (%)	52.2±14	48±10.79
sTREM-1 (pg/ml)	110 ± 18	125±28

Discussion

Despite significant progress in critical care, sepsis continues to show disproportionately high rates of mortality. [1] Delayed diagnosis, even in tertiary hospital centres, consists one of the main reasons for this pitfall. [3] In the absence of sufficient biological markers, the clinician is forced to support the diagnosis of sepsis mainly on clinical grounds (excluding the measurement of white blood cells), which makes it doubtful, since the SIRS criteria have ambiguous diagnostic performance. [4] Furthermore, other non infectious causes of SIRS, such as SLE or RA mandate different treatment strategies and management could be urgent as well. The long incubation period and modest sensitivity of blood cultures hinders a rapid final diagnosis. [5] Therefore, the need for indicators that can be used in daily clinical practice for the diagnosis or exclusion of sepsis is imperative. Several studies have evaluated the reliability of TREM-1 to diagnose infection in patients with different underlying diseases; most of them reported that it could be used as a marker to discriminate between sepsis and other causes of SIRS. [22, 23, 32] No previous study, however, has compared serum levels of TREM-1 in sepsis and autoimmune systemic inflammatory diseases, like SLE and RA.

The present study aimed to evaluate mTREM-1 and sTREM-1 in two different conditions —autoimmune SIRS and sepsis— and to determine whether these markers might be used to discriminate between the two entities.

In sepsis, mTREM-1 and sTREM-1 levels were significantly increased compared to active autoimmune patients and healthy controls; in patients with autoimmune SIRS, TREM-1 was, in turn, elevated in relation to healthy controls. To evaluate the weight of the clinical implication of sTREM-1 for differentiating sepsis from autoimmune diseases, we set the cut-off value for sTREM-1 at 100 pg/ml, with sensitivity of 72% and specificity of 99%. [32]

It seems that septic and autoimmune inflammation differs quantitatively regarding TREM-1 induction. This might be due to the different and more potent initiators (PAMPs or DAMPs) of the immune activation when it is induced against infectious agents. It could be considered that the magnitude of inflammatory reaction is augmented and more sustained in septic patients compared to autoimmune diseases. Furthermore, the disproportionate levels of CRP in SLE flares suggest that different immune pathways may be activated or inhibited in autoimmune inflammation. Although it is ambiguous if TREM-1 expression differs significantly between sepsis and other sterile causes of SIRS, there is a significant difference between sepsis and autoimmune SIRS. If there is discrepancy, specifically, between infectious and autoimmune SIRS (due to differences in antigenicity), larger studies need to be done, since few have investigated TREM-1 in autoimmunity. [38, 39, 40, 41]

Regarding RA, to our knowledge, there are no published studies evaluating sTREM-1 in serum; however, high levels of sTREM-1 in synovial fluid were reported by Kuai et al. [42] Furthermore, Collins et al. demonstrated that sTREM-1 concentrations in the synovial fluid were similar in septic arthritis and RA, but measurements were confined to local, articular expression.[41] Although one could expect that these findings could be reflected in peripheral blood, we found that this is not the case. Based on our study, the serum levels of TREM-1 are lower in patients with RA compared to septic patients. Local and peripheral levels of an inflammatory marker could be different, something usual in systemic autoimmune diseases. Probably, differences between serum and body fluids derived from the site of inflammation could be explained by the sequestration of neutrophils and macrophages taken place in situ, accompanied by forced circulation of naive cells, not yet activated. Soluble immune receptors in RA could concentrate in high amounts in synovium accompanied by a moderate increase in blood.

Regarding mTREM-1, we found a three-fold increase of its expression on CD14+ monocytes in sepsis compared to healthy controls, as other authors reported. [12, 24, 44] Knapp et al. demonstrated that mTREM-1 on macrophages was increased when healthy volunteers received an injection of LPS, with a dose- and time–dependent manner, both in vivo and in vitro. [45]

Additionally, TREM-1 expression was higher in septic rather than autoimmune patients. Presently, TREM-1 expression was compared between sepsis and sterile systemic inflammation caused by traumatic tissue damage.[43] Ferat-Osorio et al. described an increase of mTREM-1 in sepsis and in non-infectious SIRS, at the same levels. [38] This study included only surgical patients postoperatively and its conclusions could not be transferred in autoimmune patients. This discrepancy gives a clue to hypothesize that the expression of an immune receptor depends upon multiple parameters acting in a dynamic inflammatory milieu. Autoimmune and traumatic systemic inflammation could differ regarding the mechanisms of innate and adaptive immunity involved.

The levels of TREM-1 on peripheral monocytes and serum in autoimmune patients raise questions on the inflammatory pathways involved in RA and SLE. Apparently, the inflammatory reaction is not equally potent to augment TREM-1 expression at the same levels as sepsis provokes. However, its levels are well above the normal values, a finding that comes in agreement with previous studies. Molad et al. reported ten times higher sTREM-1 levels in SLE patients than normal controls.[39] Herein, we confirmed a statistically significant raise in serum sTREM-1 in SLE in comparison to healthy controls; however, the role of TREM-1 as a possible biomarker in autoimmunity warrants further investigation. Indeed, TREM-1 expression depends on the activation of several TLRs or NOD-like receptors, and besides PAMPs, many DAMPs (alarmins, such as high-mobility group box nuclear protein, heat shock proteins and free cyclic AMP) may trigger autoimmune inflammatory reactions through these receptors.

Next, we also divided sepsis patients in two subgroups depending on the presence of organ dysfunction and septic shock. We found no correlation of TREM-1 levels, membrane or soluble, to the severity of sepsis. Latour-Perez et al. conducted a cohort study finding that sTREM-1 was only marginally higher in patients with severe sepsis. [46] On the contrary, several studies have reported a positive predictive value for sTREM-1 regarding sepsis severity and mortality. [44, 45, 46] Poukoulidou et al. suggested that TREM-1 alterations upon transition from uncomplicated sepsis to septic shock were dependent on the type of infection and the causative pathogen. Additionally, mTREM-1 expression was altered at various stages of sepsis. [44] These data could explain the lack of agreement observed in clinical studies with dissimilarly designed protocols.

Furthermore, we found that there is a strong correlation between mTREM-1 and sTREM-1 levels in severe sepsis group but not in uncomplicated septic patients. Few studies, that measured mTREM-1 and sTERM-1 simultaneously, have reported different patterns of TREM-1 expression, regarding the correlation of mTREM-1 and sTREM-1 levels. [12, 27, 46] We speculate that the kinetics of mTREM-1 expression and its cleavage is altered as sepsis progress and an internal feed-back loop of regulation between mTREM-1 and sTREM-1 could be reinforced as sepsis deteriorates. The mechanisms of this regulation have not been elucidated yet.

The limitations of this study are the small number of patients, especially autoimmune patients due to the rare incidence of SIRS in these diseases. Patients with two distinct diseases were studied although our results do not demonstrate great differences in these parameters between SLE and RA. Secondly, autoimmune patients were not sex-matched to septic patients, although no gender-related difference in TREM-1 expression has been reported.

In conclusion, we can support that membrane bound and soluble TREM-1 is elevated in both septic and aseptic inflammation. In sepsis, its elevation may be more pronounced, like other biomarkers such as CRP, which is usually higher in sepsis rather than in RA or SLE, but a cut-off value has not been yet determined. From the immunological point of view, these patterns of TREM-1 expression could be explained by the different patterns of PRR activation in sepsis and autoimmune inflammation. TREM-1 may be useful for discrimination of infectious from non-infectious SIRS causes. [48, 49, 50] Our results are in accordance with other reports in the literature and the recent meta-analysis. [35] TREM-1 could be comparable to PCT, but the number of available studies for sTREM-1 is still low; its role in the diagnosis of sepsis needs to be clarified. The diagnostic accuracy of TREM-1 in autoimmune diseases, such as RA and SLE, remains an open question. How the alterations in mTREM-1 and/or sTREM-1 could predict the course of an inflammatory systemic disease could be a topic for future research.

References

[1] Martin GS, Mannino DM, Eaton S, Moss M. The epidemiology of sepsis in the United States from 1979 through 2000. *N. Engl. J. Med.* 2003; 348: 1546-54.

[2] Engel C, Brunkhorst FM. Epidemiology of sepsis in Germany: results from a national prospective multicenter study. *Intensive Care Med.* 2007; 33: 606-18.

[3] Daniels R. Surviving the first hours in sepsis: getting the basics right. *J. Antimicrob Chemotherapy* 2011; 66 (suppl 2).

[4] Dellinger RP, Levy MM. Surviving Sepsis Campaign: international guidelines for management of severe sepsis and septic shock (2012). *Intensive Care Med.* 2013; 39: 165-228.

[5] Jaimes F, Garces J. The systemic inflammatory response syndrome (SIRS) to identify infected patients in the emergency room. Intensive *Care Med.* 2003; 29: 1368-71.

[6] Nyström PO. The systemic inflammatory response syndrome: definitions and aetiology. *J. Antimicrob. Chemother* 1998; 41 (suppl 1): 1-7.

[7] Waheeda Nargis**,** Md Ibrahim**,** Borhan Uddin Ahamed**.** Procalcitonin versus C-reactive protein: Usefulness as biomarker of sepsis in ICU patient. *Int. J. Crit. Ill. Injury Sci.* 2014; 4: 195-9.

[8] Bloos F, Reinhart K. Rapid diagnosis of sepsis. *Virulence* 2014; 5: 154-60.

[9] Honore PM, Jacobs R, De Waele E, Spapen HD. Biomarkers to detect sepsis: a "burning" issue but still a long way to go. *Crit. Care Med.* 2014; 42: 2137.

[10] Pierrakos C, Vincent JL. Sepsis biomarkers: a review. *Crit. Care.* 2010; 14: R15.

[11] Lee SH, Chan RC, Wu JY, Chen HW, Chang SS, Lee CC. Diagnostic value of procalcitonin for bacterial infection in elderly patients - a systematic review and meta-analysis. *Int. J. Clin. Pract.* 2013; 67: 1350-7.

[12] Lemarié J, Barraud D, Gibot S. Host Response Biomarkers in Sepsis: Overview on sTREM-1 *Detection. Methods Mol. Biol.* 2015; 1237: 225-39.

[13] Simonsen KA, Anderson-Berry AL, Delair SF, Davies HD. Early-onset neonatal sepsis. *Clin. Microbiol. Rev.* 2014; 27: 21-47.

[14] Gros A, Roussel M, Sauvadet E et al. The sensitivity of neutrophil CD64 expression as a biomarker of bacterial infection is low in critically ill patients. *Intensive Care Med.* 2012; 38: 445–52.

[15] Gibot S, Massin F, Le Renard P, Béné MC, Faure GC, Bollaert PE, Levy B. Surface and soluble triggering receptor expressed on myeloid cells-1: expression patterns in murine sepsis. *Crit. Care Med.* 2005; 33: 1787-93.

[16] Colonna M, Facchetti F. TREM-1 (triggering receptor expressed on myeloid cells): a new player in acute inflammatory responses. *J. Infect. Dis.* 2003; 187 (Suppl 2): S397-401.

[17] Arts RJ, Joosten LA, van der Meer JW, Netea MG. TREM-1: intracellular signalling pathways and interaction with pattern recognition receptors. *J. Leukoc. Biol.* 2013; 93: 209-15.

[18] Pelham CJ, Pandya AN, Agrawal DK. Triggering receptor expressed on myeloid cells receptor family modulators: a patent review. *Expert Opin. Ther Pat* 2014; 1: 1-13.

[19] Tsujimoto H, Ono S, Efron PA, Scumpia PO, Moldawer LL, Mochizuki H. Role of Toll-like receptors in the development of sepsis. *Shock* 2008; 29: 315-21.

[20] Bostanci N, Thurnheer T, Belibasakis GN. Involvement of the TREM-1/DAP12 pathway in the innate immune responses to Porphyromonas gingivalis. *Mol. Immunol.* 201; 49: 387-94.

[21] Luo L, Zhou Q, Chen XJ, Qin SM, Ma WL, Shi HZ. Effects of the TREM-1 pathway modulation during empyema in rats. *Chin. Med. J.* (Engl) 2010; 123: 1561-5.

[22] Gibot S, Alauzet C, Massin F, Sennoune N, Faure GC, Béné MC, Lozniewski A, Bollaert PE, Lévy B. Modulation of the triggering receptor expressed on myeloid cells-1 pathway during pneumonia in rats. *J. Infect. Dis.* 2006; 194: 975-83.

[23] Gibot S, Aurélie C. Soluble Triggering Receptor Expressed on Myeloid Cells and the Diagnosis of Pneumonia. *N. Engl. J. Med.* 2004; 350: 451-8.

[24] Ubagai T, Nakano R, Kikuchi H, Ono Y. Gene expression analysis of TREM1 and GRK2 in polymorphonuclear leukocytes as the surrogate biomarkers of acute bacterial infections. *Int. J. Med. Sci.* 2014; 11: 215-21.

[25] Determann RM, Achouiti AA, El Solh AA, Bresser P, Vijfhuizen J, Spronk PE, Schultz MJ. Infectious pleural effusions can be identified by sTREM-1 levels. *Respir. Med.* 2010; 104: 310-5.

[26] Gibot S, Cravoisy A, Dupays R, Barraud D, Nace L, Levy B, Bollaert PE. Combined measurement of procalcitonin and soluble TREM-1 in the diagnosis of nosocomial sepsis. *Scand. J. Infect. Dis.* 2007; 39: 604-8.

[27] Oku R, Oda S, Nakada TA, Sadahiro T, Nakamura M, Hirayama Y, Abe R, Tateishi Y, Ito M, Iseki T, Hirasawa H. Differential pattern of cell-surface and soluble TREM-1 between sepsis and SIRS. *Cytokine* 2013; 61: 112-7.

[28] Park JJ, Cheon JH, Kim BY, Kim DH, Kim ES, Kim TI, Lee KR, Kim WH. Correlation of serum-soluble triggering receptor expressed on myeloid cells-1 with clinical disease activity in inflammatory bowel disease. *Dig. Dis. Sci.* 2009; 54: 1525-31.

[29] Bingold T, Pullmann B, Sartorius S, Geiger EV, Marzi I, Zacharowski K et al. Soluble triggering receptor on myeloid cells-1 is expressed in the course of non infectious inflammation after traumatic lung contusion: a prospective cohort study. *Critical Care* 2011; 15: R115.

[30] Prucha M, Zazula R, Muller M, Hyanek T, Dostal M, Sedlackova L. TREM-1 expression on monocytes is not a parameter specific for infectious etiology of Systematic Inflammatory Response Syndrome. *Prague Medical Report* 2011. 112: 205-21.

[31] Bopp C, Hofer S, Bouchon A et al. Soluble TREM-1 is not suitable for distinguishing between systemic inflammatory response syndrome and sepsis survivors and non survivors in the early stage of acute inflammation. *Eur. J. Anaesthesiol* 2009; 26: 504-7.

[32] Su L, Han B, Liu C et al. Value of soluble TREM-1, procalcitonin, and C-reactive protein serum levels as biomarkers for detecting bacteremia among sepsis patients with new fever in intensive care units: a prospective cohort study. *BMC Infect Dis* 2012; 12: 157.

[33] Latour-Pérez J, Alcalá-López A, García-García MA et al. Diagnostic accuracy of sTREM-1 to identify infection in critically ill patients with systemic inflammatory response syndrome. *Clin. Biochem.* 2010; 43: 720–4.

[34] Gibot S, Benet CM, Noel R et al. Combination Biomarkers to Diagnose Sepsis in the Critically Ill Patient. *Am. J. Respir. Crit. Care Med.* 2012; 186: 65–71.

[35] Wu Y, Wang F, Fan X, Bao R, Bo L, Li J, Deng X. Accuracy of plasma sTREM-1 for sepsis diagnosis in systemic inflammatory patients: a systematic review and meta-analysis. *Critical Care*. 2012; 16: R229.

[36] Aletaha D, Neogi T, Silman AJ, Funovits J, Felson DT, Bingham C et al. 2010 rheumatoid arthritis classification criteria: an American College of

Rheumatology/European League Against Rheumatism collaborative initiative. *Arthritis. Rheum.* 2010; 62: 2569–81.

[37] Hochberg MC. Updating the American College of Rheumatology revised criteria for the classification of systemic lupus erythematosus. *Arthritis. Rheum.* 1997; 40: 1725.

[38] Ferat-Osorio E, Esquivel-Callejas N, Wong-Baeza I, Aduna-Vicente R, Arriaga-Pizano L et al. The increased expression of TREM-1 on monocytes is associated with infectious and noninfectious inflammatory processes. *J. Surg. Res.* 2008; 150: 110-7.

[39] Molad Y, Pokroy-Shapira E, Kaptzan T, Monselise A, Shalita-Chesner M, Monselise Y. Serum soluble triggering receptor on myeloid cells-1 (sTREM-1) is elevated in systemic lupus erythematosus but does not distinguish between lupus alone and concurrent infection. *Inflammation* 2013; 3: 1519-24.

[40] Kamei K, Yasuda T, Ueda T, Qiang F, Takeyama Y, Shiozaki H. Role of triggering receptor expressed on myeloid cells-1 in experimental severe acute pancreatitis. *J. Hepatobiliary Pancreat Sci.* 2010; 17: 305-12.

[41] Collins CE, La DT, Yang HT, Massin F, Gibot S, Faure G, Stohl W. Elevated synovial expression of triggering receptor expressed on myeloid cells-1 in patients with septic arthritis or rheumatoid arthritis. *Ann. Rheum. Dis.* 2009; 68: 1768-74.

[42] Kuai J, Gregory B, Hill A, Pittman DD, Feldman JL, Brown T et al. TREM-1 expression is increased in the synovium of rheumatoid arthritis patients and induces the expression of pro-inflammatory cytokines. *Rheumatology* (Oxford) 2009; 48: 1352-8.

[43] Gibot S, Le Renard PE, Bollaert-Bouchon A, Facchetti F, Weigand MA, Colonna M. TREM-1 amplifies inflammation and is a crucial mediator of septic shock. *Nature* 2001; 410: 1103-7.

[44] Latour-Pérez J, Alcala-Lopez A, Garcia-Garcia MA, Sanchez-Hernandez JF, Abad-Terrado C, Viedma-Contreras JA et al. Prognostic value of the sTREM-1 plasma values in patients with sepsis: a cohort study. *Med. Intensiva* 2010; 34: 231-6.

[45] Gibot S, Le Renard PE, Bollaert PE, Kolopp-Sarda MN, Bene MC et al. Surface triggering receptor expressed on myeloid cells-1 expression patterns in septic shock. *Intensive Care Med.* 2005; 31: 594-7.

[46] Poukoulidou T, Spyridaki A, Mihailidou I, Kopterides P, Pistiki A, Alexiou Z et al. TREM-1 expression on neutrophils and monocytes of

septic patients: relation to the underlying infection and the implicated pathogen. *BMC Infect. Dis.* 2011; 11: 309.

[47] Knapp S, Gibot S, de Vos A, Versteeg HH, Colonna M, van der Poll T. Cutting edge: expression patterns of surface and soluble triggering receptor expressed on myeloid cells-1 in human endotoxemia. *J. Immunol.* 2004; 173: 7131-4.

[48] Wong-Baeza I, Gonzalez-Roldan N, Ferat-Osorio E, Esquivel-Callejas N, Aduna-Vicente R, Arriaga-Pizano L et al. Triggering receptor expressed on myeloid cells (TREM-1) is regulated post-transcriptionally and its ligand is present in the sera of some septic patients. *Clin. Exp. Immunol.* 2006; 145: 448-55.

[49] Stein M, Schachter-Davidov A, Babai I, Tasher D, Somekh E. The Accuracy of C-Reactive Protein, Procalcitonin, and s-TREM-1 in the Prediction of Serious Bacterial Infection in Neonates. *Clin. Pediatr.* (Phila) 2014; Oct 7: PMID: 25294884.

[50] Sandquist M, Wong HR. Biomarkers of sepsis and their potential value in diagnosis, prognosis and treatment. *Expert Rev. Clin. Immunol.* 2014; 10: 1349-56.

In: Septic Shock
Editor: Benedict Graver
ISBN: 978-1-63463-916-3

Chapter V

Bridging Danger Signals from within and without: High Mobility Group Box 1

Joo Guan Yeo,[1] Jing Yao Leong,[2] and Jan Hau Lee[1,2*]

[1]Department of Pediatrics Subspecialities, Children's Intensive Care Unit, KK Women's and Children's Hospital, Singapore

[2]Sing Health Translational Immunology and Inflammation Centre, The Academia, Singapore

Abstract

Multicellular organisms detect danger signals from tissue injury through pattern recognition receptors. These signals serve to initiate the appropriate immune responses that will lead to timely removal of its causative source to prevent further tissue damage. These danger signals, collectively known as damage associated molecular patterns (DAMPs), can be divided into exogenous pathogen associated molecular patterns and endogenous alarmins. In health, DAMPs work in an orchestrated

* Correspondence to: Jan Hau Lee, Children's Intensive Care Unit, KK Women's and Children's Hospital, 100 Bukit Timah Road, Singapore 229899, Tel.: +65 63926347, Fax: +65 62917923, e-mail: lee.jan.hau@kkh.com.sg

appropriate manner leading to the clearance of the insult. Dysregulation of DAMPs in disease state can lead to an inappropriate systemic inflammatory response syndrome. Here, we review high mobility group box 1 (HMGB1), a DAMP of significant relevance to the continual propagation of sepsis-induced inflammation. HMGB1, a ubiquitous nuclear protein, released after infection, tissue injury and cell death has been identified as a key late mediator of sepsis-related death in murine models. Unlike early inflammatory mediators where biological pathways have already been activated upon diagnosis of sepsis, HMGB1's delayed role potentially opens a therapeutic window to antagonize its effects. HMGB1's known biological functions and mechanism in which it mediates inflammation, clinical relevance as revealed in human sepsis cohorts and current novel experimental therapeutic intervention are discussed in this review.

Keywords: Damage associated molecular patterns, high mobility group box 1, sepsis

Abbreviations

α7nAChR, α7 nicotinic acetylcholine receptor
CpG-ODN, CpG oligodeoxynucleotides
CLP, cecal ligation and perforation
DAMPs, damage associated molecular patterns
DNA, deoxyribonucleic acid
ELISA, enzyme linked immunosorbent assay
HMGB1, high mobility group box 1
HSP, heat shock proteins; IFN, interferon; IL, interleukin
LPS, lipopolysaccharide
NF-κB, nuclear factor kappa-light-chain-enhancer of activated B cells
NLS, nuclear localising signals
PAMPs, pathogen associated molecular patterns
PBMCs, peripheral blood mononuclear cells
PRR, pattern recognition receptors
RAGE, receptor for advanced glycation end-products
RNA, ribonucleic acid
ROS, reactive oxygen species
siRNA, small interfering RNA

TLRs, Toll-like receptors
TNF, tumor necrosis factor

Introduction

Sepsis remains an important cause of mortality and morbidity despite modern medical care and antibiotic therapy [1, 2]. In its most life-threatening form with organ failure, severe sepsis has an estimated population incidence of 300 per 100,000 and a mortality of between 10 to 40% [2]. In the quest of improving clinical outcome, interest has been focused primarily on the inflammatory mediators (such as tumor necrosis factor (TNF)-α, interleukin (IL)-1β and IL-6) with the aim of exploring targeted biological therapy. In septic patients, increasing levels of these inflammatory mediators strongly correlated with mortality [3]. Although biologics have been proven to be an extremely useful arsenal against autoimmune sterile inflammation, results in septic patients have been disappointing, with inhibition of cytokines such as TNF-α and IL-1β showing no improvement in survival rates [4, 5]. The failure of these clinical trials highlights the possibility that other late mediators of the infective inflammatory process may play a critical role in causing end organ injury and lethality. High mobility group box 1 (HMGB1), an alarmin (i.e., endogenous damage associated molecular pattern (DAMP)), is one example of a late mediator [6]. HMGB1 is released by the host after it senses the presence of an invading pathogen and is responsible for the propagation of the immune response from within. Prior to the discovery of its role in inflammation, HMGB1 was viewed as a ubiquitous structural DNA binding protein, present in all nucleated cells [7, 8]. In murine endotoxemia model, systemic HMGB1 release was delayed (detectable at 8 hours) and plateaued from 16 to 32 hours after lipopolysaccharide (LPS) injection [6]. Antagonism with anti-HMGB1 antibodies protected mice from death and when mice were injected with recombinant HMGB1 alone, the endotoxin lethality was recapitulated even in the absence of LPS and other pro-inflammatory cytokines. This proves that HMGB1 is an important downstream mediator of endotoxemia. The fact that HMGB1 is secreted late in sepsis and inhibition of HMGB1 alone appears to be sufficient to protect against endotoxin lethality without the need to inhibit other upstream components/cytokines makes it a promising therapeutic target in severe sepsis. In this review, we aim to provide an overview of the DAMPs with an eventual focus on HMGB1. The following areas on HMGB1 will be covered: 1) structure and relevant post-translational modifications; 2) interaction and complex formation with other DAMPs; 3) mechanisms of action; 4) current novel experimental therapeutic intervention in animals/ humans; and 5) clinical relevance in human sepsis cohorts.

DAMPs: Signature of Danger

The innate immune system provides a rapid, poly-specific response that is able to discriminate self from non-self through recognition of pathogen associated molecular patterns (PAMPs) by host pattern recognition receptors (PRRs) [9]. Collectively, PAMPs are highly conserved and common constituents of a large number of pathogenic microbes such as LPS, mannans, glycans, bacterial double-stranded deoxyribonucleic acid (DNA) and ribonucleic acid (RNA). As these PAMPSs are not found in the host, discrimination from self is possible. PAMPs are important in initiating the immune response for pathogens clearance before significant injuries to the host can occur.

Danger signals, known as alarmins, can also arise internally within the host from sterile injuries [10]. Alarmins are normally hidden from recognition by the immune system by being sequestered within the intracellular component. However, in pathological states such as trauma and ischemia, these molecules can be released by damaged cells [11]. Like PAMPs, alarmins can elicit an immune response, which in health, is important for injury resolution and repair of the damaged tissue [12]. Important examples of alarmins include HMGB1, S100 proteins and heat shock proteins (HSP) [10, 11, 13]. Collectively, alarmins (endogenous danger signals) and PAMPs (exogenous pathogen related danger signals) are known as DAMPs [10]. They function to eliminate the source of the danger signals (DAMPs) by various effector mechanisms mediated through the PRRs to re-establish homeostasis. However, when dysregulated, exaggerated and persistent inflammatory response can occur to cause host tissue injuries.

The PRRs, which provides the initial recognition that will lead to the activation of downstream effector response, can be functionally divided into 3 classes: 1) secreted, 2) endocytic, and 3) signaling [14]. Secreted PRRs (e.g., ficolins and mannose binding lectins) are important in the complement system [15-17]. Their main roles include opsonisation of microbes/damaged cells for removal via phagocytosis through complement receptors and activation of the complement system to generate more opsonins, anaphylatoxins for immune cells recruitment and membrane attack complexes formation with bacterial lysis [15, 16, 18, 19]. Endocytic PRRs are found on surfaces of phagocytes (e.g., macrophages) allowing for the uptake of microbes/damaged cells for its delivery to the lysosomes for subsequent destruction [14, 16]. Signaling PRRs are typified by the toll-like receptors (TLRs) which when ligated will lead to downstream signaling with activation of immune response genes leading to the release of cytokines (TNF-α, IL-6), chemokines and increase expression of surface co-stimulatory molecules [20-22].

Unlike most of the alarmins which mediates only sterile inflammation, HMGB1's immunological role appears to straddle both infective and non-infective inflammation [23, 24]. In addition, HMGB1 appears to work in a coordinated, orchestrated manner with PAMPs in sepsis where LPS initiates the initial immune response that will lead to subsequent release of HMGB1 that culminates in endotoxin lethality in mice [6].

HMGB1 Structure and Post-Translational Modifications

HMGB1 is a relatively small protein consisting of 215 amino acid residues (Figure 1A). Although small, it has distinct segments that have different biological activities (Figure 1B). Other than its primary structure, oxidation-reduction, acetylation and phosphorylation (post-translational modifications) of HMGB1 are also important in influencing its function as an alarmin [25-29]. HMGB1 consists of 3 domains: 2 positively charged DNA-binding domains (HMG boxes A and B) and an acidic tail containing aspartic and glutamic acids (Figure 1A) [13]. It contains 43 lysine residues, of which there are 2 predominant lysine clusters within the 2 nuclear localising signals (NLSs) (NLS1 = amino acids 28 to 44; NLS2 = amino acids 179180 to 185). The acetylation status of the NLSs will determine the direction of the nucleocytoplasmic shuttling and eventual extracellular secretion [26]. In addition, HMGB1 contains 3 highly conserved cysteines that are readily oxidized (box A position 23 and 45, box B position 106) (Figure 1A).

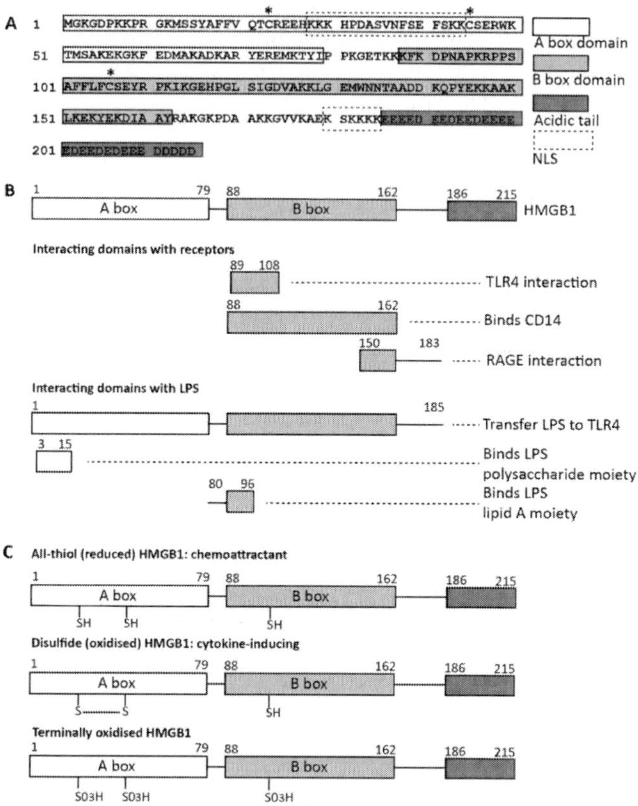

Figure 1. Structure and functional domains of HMGB1. A. A linear representation of HMGB1 with the amino acid residues (denoted by its single letter code, e.g., A: alanine) that constitutes its A-box, B-box and acidic tail. The 2 NLSs contains lysine (K) residues that when acetylated, will accumulate in the cytosol. The conserved cysteine residues at position 23, 45 and 106 are marked with an asterisk (*). B. Interacting regions of HMGB1 with receptor for advanced glycation end-products (RAGE), TLR4, CD14 and LPS. HMGB1 interaction with TLR4 occurs at position 89 to 108. This is the minimum region requires to recapitulate the pro-inflammatory activity of full length HMGB1. RAGE interacts with HMGB1 from position 150 to 183 of B-box and part of the linker region to the acidic tail. HMGB1 interaction with LPS is well defined. The A and B boxes must be in continuity for HMGB1 to be able to transfer LPS to CD14 that will result in TLR4 activation. The regions that interact with the LPS polysaccharide and lipid A moieties have been defined through truncation studies. C. HMGB1 redox status and activity. Mutually exclusive redox forms of HMGB1 promote different immunological activities: reduced cysteines make HMGB1 a chemoattractant, a disulfide bond between the cysteine residues at position 23 and 45 with a thiol group at cysteine 106 makes it pro-inflammatory, and terminal oxidation of all its cysteines to sulfonates by reactive oxygen species (ROS) abrogates both activities.

Extracellular HMGB1 is derived mainly from two pathways: 1) active secretion from activated macrophages [6], neutrophils [30] , dendritic cells [31], plasmacytiod dendritic cells [32], and activated natural killer cells [33] and 2) passive release from primary or secondary necrotic cells (late apoptotic cells) [34, 35]. HMGB1 lacks a secretory signal peptide within its sequence. Active secretion occurs through three main pathways: 1) hyperacetylation of HMGB1 lysine (K) residues within its 2 NLSs leads to its accumulation in secretory lysosomes [26]; 2) phosphorylation of its serine (S) residues [36]; and 3) mono-methylation on lysine (K) 42 in neutrophils [30]. The eventual active secretionrelease is mediated via a vesicle-mediate secretory pathway triggered by lysophosphatidylcholine [27].

Other than affecting its cellular localisation, there is accumulating evidence that post-translation modifications of HMGB1 can influence its ability to mediate various immunological processes [37, 38]. Oxidation-reduction is the most important in this aspect.

HMGB1 can exist in 3 different redox forms (Figure 1C). The chemoattractant reduced HMGB1 (all-thiol-HMGB1) has its 3 cysteine (C) residues containing a thiol group each [37]. Its ability to mediate inflammatory cells recruitment is dependent on its complex formation with the C-X-C motif chemokine ligand 12 (CXCL12) and the subsequent binding of this all-thiol-HMGB1-CXCL12 heterocomplex to the C-X-C motif chemokine receptor 4 (CXCR4) [39]. The pro-inflammatory oxidized HMGB1 (disulfide HMGB1) contains a disulfide bond between the cysteine residues at position 23 and 45 with a thiol group at cysteine residue at position 106 and is able to induce TNF-α production in macrophages [37, 38]. The critical region responsible for this proinflammatory activity is from amino acid residues 89 to 108 with the cysteine at position 106 having a thiol group (Figure 1B and C) [40, 41]. This effect is mediated by direct TLR4 ligation. Lastly, HMGB1 can also be terminally oxidized to sulfonates in the presence of high levels of reactive oxygen species (ROS) and this abrogates both its cytokine-inducing and chemoattractant activities [37]. The terminal oxidization of HMGB1 has also been shown to be able to redirect its ability from activation of the acquired immune responses toward tolerance [42].

It is likely that the 3 redox states of HMGB1 exists as a continuum, mediating different phases of healing from the initial injury with immune cells recruitment, inflammation followed by eventual resolution and repair [43]. When muscle necrosis was induced by cardiotoxin injection in mice, all-thiol HMGB1 was detected at an early time point (2 hours) with the disulfide-HMGB1 appearing later (6 hours). The all-thiol HMGB1 was likely to be passively released by the damaged cells resulting in recruitment of inflammatory cells with the formation of ROS that partially oxidized the extracellular all-thiol HMGB1 to form the pro-inflammatory disulfide HMGB1 [37]. Of note, monocytic cells when stimulated with LPS had all-thiol-HMGB1 in the intracellular compartment (nucleus and cytosol) while the extracellular supernatant contained a mixture of all-thiol-HMGB1 (chemoattractant) and disulfide-HMGB1 (pro-inflammatory) further supporting the occurrence of partial oxidation of HMGB1 by extracellular ROS after it was released [37].

These sequential changes were also observed in murine acetaminophen-induced hepatic necrosis where in active inflammation, HMGB1 was predominantly in the active disulfide form whereas during resolution and regeneration, terminally oxidized inactive HMGB1 accumulated [38]. These findings suggest a possible protective role of terminal oxidation as a negative regulatory mechanism in HMGB1 biology during persistent inflammation. Less is known about the effect of other modifications on HMGB1's immunological properties.

Thus, given the stark difference in functions of the various HMGB1 redox forms, determination of total HMGB1 in the circulation alone without the consideration of the concentration of the different redox forms is unlikely to be clinically useful.

HMGB1 Heterocomplex Formation with Other Danger Signals

Another important consideration in HMGB1's biological activity is its ability to interact with other endogenous and exogenous danger signals [44]. HMGB1 has an adjuvant-like effect in enhancing/synergizing inflammatory effects of these danger signals. HMGB1 has been demonstrated to interact with Pam3CSK4 (a synthetic triacylated lipoprotein and TLR1/2 ligand), LPS (TLR4 ligand), nucleosome complexes, CpG oligodeoxynucleotides (CpG-ODNs) (TLR9 ligand), DNA-containing immune complexes (formed from autoantibodies and autoantigens), and IL-1β [28, 44-49]. Interacting partners with HMGB1 and the biological effects they mediate are summarized in Table 1.

HMGB1's synergistic effect with LPS, Pam3CSK4, CpG-ODN and IL-1β in stimulating human peripheral blood mononuclear cells' (PBMCs') IL-6 production appears to be independent of HMGB1's post-translational modifications [44].

Table 1. HMGB1 interacting partners and their biological effects

Type of signals	Interacting partners	Biological effects	Refs
PAMPs	CpG-ODN (type A)	HMGB1 bound to CpG-ODN (type A) and stimulated interferon (IFN)-α production in a TLR9 and RAGE dependent manner in mouse plasmacytiod dendritic cells.	[46]
	CpG-ODN (type B)	HMGB1 interacted with TLR9 in the endoplasmic reticulum Golgi intermediate compartment and hastened TLR9 redistribution to early endosomes in response to CpG-ODN leading to secretion of IL-6, IL-12 and TNF-α by mouse bone marrow derived dendritic cells.	[45]
	LPS	HMGB1 caused disaggregation of LPS from micelle and transferred it to CD14 to initiate TLR4 mediated response. HMGB1 had a synergistic effect with LPS in stimulating TNF-α production in human PBMCs and peripheral blood monocytes.	[28]
	LPS, Pam3CSK4, and CpG ODN (type B)	HMGB1 synergized with its partners to stimulate IL-6 production in cultured human PBMCs.	[44]
Alarmins	Systemic lupus erythematosus immune complexes	The induction of genes encoding type 1 IFN in PBMCs by systemic lupus erythematosus immune complexes was dependent on the presence of HMGB1 and RAGE.	[46]
	Nucleosomes (DNA-histones complex)	HMGB1-containing nucleosomes from apoptotic cells induced secretion of IL-1β, IL-6 and TNF-α from human macrophages and expression of co-stimulatory molecules from human monocyte derived dendritic cells. HMGB1-containing nucleosomes induced anti-dsDNA and antihistone IgG in a TLR2 dependent manner.	[47]
	IL-1β	HMGB1 synergized with IL-1β to stimulate IL-6 production in cultured human PBMCs.	[44]
	DNA-containing immune complexes	Requirement of HMGB1 in the induction of anti-dsDNA antibody production by cultured systemic lupus erythematosus patient's PBMCs through a TLR2 dependent pathway.	[49]
Others	CXCL12 (chemokine)	Heterocomplex formation of all-thio (oxidized) HMGB1 with CXCL12 leading to binding to CXCR4 (chemokine receptor) with inflammatory cells recruitment.	[39]

The significance of HMGB1 ability to complex with many different other danger signals leads to the inability of enzyme linked immunosorbent assay (ELISA) to accurately determine its true concentration in the serum/plasma due to the steric hindrance or epitope masking posed by its binding partners preventing recognition by capture antibody [50]. This compounds the problem that is already present as a result of different HMGB1 post-translational modifications mentioned previously.

Mechanism of Action

Receptors that mediate HMGB1 inflammatory responses include receptor for advanced glycation end-products (RAGE), TLR2, TLR4, TLR9 and CD24-Siglec-10 (Siglec-G in mice) [51-55]. The entire spectrum of HMGB1 receptors mediates inflammatory responses with the exception of CD24-Siglec-10 [55]. CD24-Siglec-10 appears to selectively repress inflammatory response to proteins released by damaged cells (i.e., endogenous danger signals such as HMGB1, HSP70 and HSP90) but not to ligands of bacterial origin (i.e., PAMP such as LPS).

As many of the inflammatory responses are mediated by HMGB1 in complexes with DAMPs (IL-1β, LPS, CpG-ODN, and Pam3CSK4), nucleosomes or autoantibodies-autoantigens immune complexes, direct HMGB1-receptor interaction and signaling may not be necessary. These HMGB1-partner molecule complexes are likely to signal through the partner molecule's receptors (Table 1) [56].

Direct HMGB1-receptor binding has only been demonstrated with RAGE and TLR4 with the corresponding binding regions on HMGB1 elucidated [41, 57].

RAGE is a multi-ligands receptor implicated in a wide variety of acute and chronic inflammatory diseases [58]. Like the TLR, it can be considered as a PRR and is able to bind to DAMPs such as HMGB1 and S100 proteins. RAGE had been shown to be important in mediating HMGB1 pro-inflammatory effects in mouse macrophages [51].

HMGB1 is able to exert its cytokine-like activity either alone or in synergism with LPS (Figure 1B and C) [25, 28]. As discussed previously, HMGB1 cytokine-like activity is dependent on its redox status: the cysteines residues at position 23 and 45 must form a disulfide bond and cysteine 106 must be in the thiol state [37, 38]. HMGB1 B-box exhibits proinflammatory functionality required for the stimulation of macrophages cytokines release, with the critical region spanning from position 89 to 108 [40]. Within this region, the cysteine 106 residue is critical for HMGB1 binding to TLR4 and mutation of this residue to alanine abrogated its binding to TLR4, thereby preventing cytokine release from macrophages [41].

With LPS, HMGB1 augments its pro-inflammatory activity in a synergistic manner. HMGB1 binds to LPS and facilitates its transfer to CD14 leading to TLR4 ligation and enhancement of TNF-α production by human monocytes [28].

This activity is dependent on the presence of both the A and B HMG boxes but not the acidic tail [28]. The regions important for this activity have been further elucidated: HMGB1 amino acid residues position 3 to 15 (within A box) and 80 to 96 (linker region and B box), are found to bind polysaccharide and lipid A moieties of LPS respectively [59]. As for the CD14 binding region, it involves region of the B-box (Figure 1B).

Targeting HMGB1 in Sepsis

The validation of the biological importance of HMGB1 in-vivo in various inflammatory diseases including sepsis has been hampered by the lethality of HMGB1 knockout due to death from severe postnatal hypoglycaemia in mice models [60]. However, recently, this limitation has been circumvented through the selective deletion of the HMGB1 gene in myeloid cells using site-specific recombinase technology as well as targeted delivery of HMGB1 small interfering RNA (siRNA) to human macrophages and dendritic cell found in humanized mice [61, 62].

In the past, HMGB1's role in infective inflammation had been mostly demonstrated indirectly through neutralizing antibodies (polyclonal and monoclonal), antagonism/sequestration (HMGB1 A-box fragment or thrombomodulin), inhibition of its release, inhibition of the HMGB1-RAGE axis and physical removal of endotoxin (that mediates HMGB1 release) through absorption (Table 2) [6, 63-73]. In terms of therapeutic targeting of HMGB1 in sepsis, the use of monoclonal and polyclonal antibodies and finally, antagonism/sequestration of HMGB1 provides most specificity. The two common severe sepsis models used are: 1) endotoxemia with LPS administration and 2) intra-abdominal polymicrobial sepsis from cecal ligation and perforation (CLP).

The targeting of HMGB1 in sepsis models using antibodies, HMGB1 A-box antagonist, or sequestration (direct binding with inactivation) has been promising. This was first described by Wang and colleagues in 1999 when they noticed the delayed release kinetics of HMGB1 (from 8 to 32 hours) as compared to other cytokines in endotoxemia mice and successfully reduced lethality with neutralizing polyclonal anti-HMGB1 treatment [6]. A consistent feature among all the studies where HMGB1 activity was antagonized was the fairly long lasting survival of up to 3 weeks (Table 2).

These results was subsequently similarly demonstrated with CLP models [64]. Pathophysiologically, this in-vivo model closely mimics that of human severe sepsis (with the presence of live bacteria and systemic inflammatory response with organ dysfunction: such as renal impairment with elevated blood urea nitrogen and creatinine). CLP is considered the gold standard for in-vivo sepsis model for pre-clinical evaluation of new treatment for severe sepsis [74]. In CLP, the increase in HMGB1 began later at 18 hours as compared to that observed in the endotoxemia model and remained persistently elevated up to 72 hours. When anti-HMGB1 was given at 24 hours after CLP, mice was rescued from lethal experimental sepsis [64]. Similar results were obtained with the antagonist, HMGB1 A-box. Of note, administration of treatment even when established signs of sepsis were present in the mice still results in clinical improvement.

The next agent that targets HMGB1 is thrombomodulin and its administration decreased murine lethality from endotoxemia [63]. Thrombomodulin binds to HMGB1 with its N-terminal lectin-like domain, hence sequestering and preventing its binding to RAGE and downstream inflammatory activity. Thrombomodulin is important as it is part of the anticoagulation pathway and its derangement is observed in sepsis-induced disseminated intravascular coagulopathy [75]. In addition, its administration was found to be safe and of potential benefit in these patients [76, 77]. However, larger randomized control trial will still be required to determine its efficacy and to define the subgroup that will benefit from it. It will also be interesting to further study whether thrombomodulin is able to sequester HMGB1 and prevents its heterocomplex formation and adjuvant like effect with other DAMPs as well as prevent its binding to TLR4.

Multiple pharmacological agents have been shown to inhibit HMGB1 release (Table 2). However, it may be difficult to attribute the observed effects to inhibition of HMGB1 release alone as other inflammatory mediators may be concurrently affected. Some of the more promising agents will be described here. Ethyl pyruvate is one such agent that is able to inhibit HMGB1 release by activated macrophages in response to LPS [73]. In addition, ethyl pyruvate is able to inhibit the signal transduction pathways, p38 mitogen-activated protein kinase and nuclear factor kappa-light-chain-enhancer of activated B cells (NF-κB), which are critical for cytokines release. In-vivo, administration of ethyl pyruvate was observed to reduce HMGB1 level and improved survival in mice with established endotoxemia or polymicrobial sepsis from CLP. As HMGB1 has been demonstrated to be a late mediator of endotoxemia lethality, it is thus likely that the improved survival is due partially to the reduction of circulating HMGB1 in addition to its inhibitory effect on the intracellular pro-inflammatory signaling cascade.

Cholinergic agonists (nicotine and acetylcholine) decreases the release of HMGB1 due to nuclear retention, inhibits the initial cytosolic translocation that is necessary for secretion [65]. This is mediated by the α7 nicotinic acetylcholine receptor (α7nAChR). Interestingly, this receptor has been utilised subsequently to silence HMGB1 through siRNA conjugated with a specific α7nAChR ligand (rabies virus glycoprotein-9R (9 arginine residues)) allowing targeted delivery of the siRNA to macrophages and dendritic cells that express the receptor [61].

This provides a specific reversible method of cell specific targeting of HMGB1 that may be of potential therapeutic use. With the use of humanized mice (immunodeficient nonobese diabetic mice transplanted with human hematopoietic cells) and the specific silencing of HMGB1 in macrophages and dendritic cells, lethality from CLP was reduced even with delayed siRNA therapy 10 hours after the surgical procedure.

Another category of agents that reduce HMGB1 secretion are the endogenous neuropeptides: vasoactive intestinal peptide, urocortin and ghrelin [70, 71]. These agents are of significance as they are believed to be part of the self-controlled anti-inflammatory mediators of the host.

Vasoactive intestinal peptide and urocortin were administered late at 12 or 24 hours after CLP in mice [71]. By then, the inflammatory cytokines (TNF-α, IL-1β, and IL-6) had already peaked (at between 6 to 12 hours), and the late administration of vasoactive intestinal peptide and urocortin were shown not to affect these cytokines level at 24 hours. In contrast, HMGB1 level was significantly reduced in both treatment. Similar results were obtained from ghrelin administration starting at 12 or 24 hours followed by maintenance dosing after CLP [70]. All the neuropeptides were shown to prevent the cytoplasmic translocation of HMGB1, a pre requisite step in its secretion.

Table 2. Therapy targeting HMGB1 in animal sepsis models

Model	Therapy	Timing	Outcome measures	References
Endotoxemia: systemic inflammatory response by LPS administration	Polyclonal anti-HMGB1	2, 12 and 36 hours after LPS.	Improved survival in mice (up to 14 days).	[6]
		2, 12 and 24 hours after LPS.	Improved survival in mice (up to 4 days).	[63]
	Antagonistic HMGB1 A-box	2, 12 and 24 hours after LPS.	Improved survival in mice (up to 14 days). Decreased end organ injuries (lower lactate dehydrogenase, blood urea nitrogen and creatinine).	[64]
	Binding/ Inactivation: Thrombomodulin	2, 12 and 24 hours after LPS.	Improved survival in mice (up to 4 days).	[63]
	Inhibition of release: Nicotine	30 minutes before LPS injection, subsequently twice per day for 3 days.	Improved survival in mice (up to 21 days).	[65]
	Ethyl pyruvate	At 4, 8, 12, 24 and 30 hours.	Improved survival in mice (up to 21 days).	[73]
	Ghrelin	At 2, 4 or 12 hours (single dose).	1) Improved survival in mice even for the delayed group of 12 hours (up to 4 days).	[70]
Live intra-abdominal polymicrobial sepsis: CLP	Anti-HMGB1 monoclonal antibody (2 clones) Epitopes: A-box amino acid residues 53 to 63 and 67 to 78.	24 hours after CLP (single dose).	Improved survival in mice (up to 14 days). Decreased end organ injuries (lower lactate dehydrogenase, blood urea nitrogen, alkaline phosphatase, aspartate transaminase, and alanine aminotransferase)	[66]

Model	Therapy	Timing	Outcome measures	References
	Polyclonal anti-HMGB1 (raised against HMGB1 B-box: amino acid residues 88 to 162.)	12 or 24 hours after CLP (maintenance twice daily for 3 days).	Improved survival in mice (up to 14 days) (but not when therapy was initiated at 36 hours after CLP).	[64]
	Polyclonal anti-HMGB1 (raised against full length HMGB1).	15 minutes after CLP (single dose).	Improved survival in rats (up to 10 days). Decrease lung tissue destruction.	[67]
	Monoclonal anti-RAGE (blocking of ligand binding to RAGE including HMGB1 but not exclusively.)	24 hours after CLP (single dose).	Improved survival in mice (up to 7 days) (but not when therapy was initiated at 36 hours after CLP). Decrease lung tissue necrosis (pathology scoring). Similar tissue bacteria concentrations (anti-RAGE and control serum).	[68]
	Antagonistic HMGB1 A-box	24 hours after CLP (maintenance twice daily for 3 days).	Improved survival in mice (up to 14 days). Decreased end organ injuries (lower lactate dehydrogenase, blood urea nitrogen and creatinine).	[64]
	Inhibition of release: Nicotine	24 hours after CLP (maintenance 3 times a day for 3 days).	Improved survival in mice (up to 21 days).	[65]
	Ethyl pyruvate	24, 30, 48 and 54 hours.	Improved survival in mice (up to 21 days).	[73]
	Low dose cisplatin	1 hour after CLP (single dose).	Improved survival in mice (up to 96 hours). Survival benefit negated when higher dose of cisplatin used. Decrease lung inflammation and damage (histology).	[69]

Table 2. (Continued)

Model	Therapy	Timing	Outcome measures	References
	Vasoactive intestinal peptideVIP and urocortin	12 or 24 hours after CLP (maintenance 8 hourly for 3 days).	1) Improved survival in mice (up to 10 days).	[71]
	Ghrelin	Starting at 12 or 24 hours after CLP (maintenance at 12, 18, 24, 36, 48, and 72 hours).	1) Improved survival in mice (up to 10 days).	[70]
	HMGB1 siRNA (targeted delivery to human macrophages and dendritic cells in immunodeficient non-obese diabetic mouse with transplanted human hematopoietic cells).	Pre-event group: 15 hours before CLP and 2 and 24 hours thereafter. Post-event group: 10, 24 and 48 hours after CLP.	Improved survival (in both groups, although lesser degree in post-event group).	[61]
	Hemoperfusion with polymyxin B-immobilized fiber.	From 3 to 6 hours post CLP.	Improved survival in piglets (short observation of 24 hours).	[72]

In addition, exogenous administration of recombinant HMGB1 reversed the therapeutic effect of all these neuropeptides at least partially, suggesting that HMGB1 was one of the mediators involved.

The last drug of interest is low dose cisplatin [69]. Cisplatin is a chemotherapeutic drug that causes DNA damage and HMGB1 has the inherent ability to bind to altered DNA structure [78].

This results results in the nuclear retention of HMGB1 and prevents its release. Although interesting, the value of this drug as an anti-HMGB1 therapeutic agent is limited as higher doses of cisplatin negates the observed survival benefit after CLP in mice [69]. In addition, the drug was administered 1 hour after CLP which would be therapeutically difficult to achieve in human sepsis.

Other than In addition to HMGB1's role in extracellular pro-inflammatory modulation, recent studies demonstrate the potential protective role of intracellular HMGB1 against endotoxemia in mice [62]. This was done with the cell specific conditional ablation of HMGB1 in the myeloid cells (including the macrophages) in mice using the Cre-LoxP system. In brief, mice with the *cre* recombinase gene inserted into the *lysozyme M* (*LysM*) locus were crossed with mice carrying the loxP flanked (floxed) *Hmgb1* gene to obtain mice carrying both the floxed *Hmgb1* and *LysM cre* genes.

As *LysM* was specifically and actively transcribed in the myeloid cells, the *cre* recombinase would also be expressed.

This resulted in the excision of the *Hmgb1* gene flanked by the LoxP sequence recognized by *cre* and complete absence of HMGB1 protein in these myeloid cells.

This circumvents the problem of a lack of HMGB1 knockout mice due to its lethality when HMGB1 is absent in all tissues.

$LysM^{Cre/+}$-$HMGB1^{f/f}$ mice were more susceptible to LPS showing decrease survival and notably specific increase in IL-1β and IL-18 (hallmark of inflammasome activation) as compared to control $LysM^{+/+}$-$HMGB1^{f/f}$ mice.

When stimulated with LPS (PAMP) and ATP (alarmin), ex-vivo macrophages from $LysM^{Cre/+}$-$HMGB1^{f/f}$ mice produced more IL-1β and IL-18 as compared to $Lys^{+/+}$-$HMGB1^{f/f}$ macrophages. This suggests that intracellular HMGB1 serves as a negative regulator of intracellular inflammasome assembly and activation.

Thus, this imparts a protective role of intracellular HMGB1 against uncontrolled inflammation from endotoxemia. This result is not in contradiction with the study by Ye and colleagues as their model uses a different system with siRNA where HMGB1 production is reduced but not completely abrogated [61].

Small amount of intracellular HMGB1 may still be present to exert its intracellular protective effect. This is an inherent property of siRNA where silencing at the level of the messenger RNA is usually incomplete and requires repeated administration of siRNA due to its degradation [79].

In addition, these two studies are also not entirely comparable due to the different sepsis models used: Ye et al. uses the CLP model while Yanai et al. uses the endotoxemia model [61, 62].

Collectively, these findings point consistently towards a pro-inflammatory role of extracellular HMGB1 whereas intracellular HMGB1 has an anti-inflammatory effect by being a negative regulator of inflammasome assembly in sepsis. All these in-vivo data suggests that blocking of the release of HMGB1 and the antagonism of its extracellular effect is of therapeutic potential in sepsis. In humans, the therapeutic potential of targeting HMGB1 in sepsis is suggested by the following observations. 1) The presence of naturally occurring anti-HMGB1 IgG that appears in patients with septic shock is significantly associated with patient survival [80]. However, as with all observational studies, the results may be confounded by other factors and attribution of causality must be done with caution. In addition, the mechanisms by which these antibodies can protect against sepsis have not been elucidated completely. 2) In patients with septic shock that respond with an increase in systolic blood pressure after hemoperfusion with polymyxin B-immobilized fiber, a statistically significant reduction in HMGB1 levels was correspondingly observed [81]. Polymyxin B functions to bind to circulating endotoxin.

Detection of HMGB1 and Correlation to Severe Sepsis Severity in Humans

In humans, HMGB1 demonstrates similar delayed release kinetics in sepsis but it is controversial whether a high level is associated with higher mortality. Out of 5 adult prospective cohort studies involving sepsis, only 3 demonstrated significant increase mortality with higher HMGB1 (Table 3) [6, 82-85]. However, the usage of different assays makes their comparison

Table 3. Quantification of HMGB1 in human sepsis cohorts

Author/Year of publication	Study type	Patients	Variable measured/Assay(s)	Controls	Outcomes
Wang H.C. et al. 1999 [6].	Prospective cohort study	25 with severe sepsis (bacteraemia and organ dysfunction). 9 gram positive, 12 gram negative and 5 un-identified.	Serum HMGB1/Western blot quantification.	8 normal controls (no detectable HMGB1)	Mortality: survivors' mean HMGB1 25.2 ng/ml. Non-survivors' mean HMGB1 83.7 ng/ml. $p < 0.05$.
Sunden- Cullberg J. et al. 2005 [82].	Prospective cohort study	26 with severe sepsis and 33 with septic shock.	Serum HMGB1 at 0, 24, 48, 96, and 144 hours/ Western blot quantification after initial preparation by two methods. Method 1: initial purification of HMGB1 from serum with heparin Sepharose beads. Method 2: concentrate obtained from the ultra-filtrate with a 100 kilo-Dalton molecular weight cut-off.	5 with sepsis	HMGB1 remained high through the study period with a value of 34 ± 76 ng/ml (mean ± standard deviation) at 144 hours. No correlation between HMGB1 and organ dysfunction score at all-time points. 28 day mortality: statistically significant lower HMGB1 (Method 1) for non-survivor (n=10) as compared to survivor (n=54). No difference (Method 2).

Table 3. (Continued)

Author/Year of publication	Study type	Patients	Variable measured/Assay(s)	Controls	Outcomes
Gibot S. et al. 2007 [83].	Prospective cross-sectional study	42 patients (62.2 ±17.4 years) (mean ± standard deviation) with septic shock. 30 out of 42 had identified pathogens, 12 gram negative and 18 gram positive.	Serum HMGB1 at day 1, 3, 7, and 14/ HMGB1 ELISA Kit II (Shino-Test Corporation, Kanagawa, Japan).	None	28 day mortality: Survivor's versus non-survivor's HMGB1 (day 1): 3.2 ng/ml (0-18.5) versus 6.2 ng/ml (2.7-18.5) (median (inter-quartile range)), $p = 0.47$. Survivor's versus non-survivor's HMGB1 (day 3): 2.7 ng/ml (0-6.0) versus 18.2 ng/ml (2.4-26.9) (median (inter-quartile range)), $p = 0.02$ (Mann-Whitney *U*- test). At a cut-off HMGB1 concentration of 4 ng/ml, odds ratio for death: 5.5 (95% confidence interval: 1.3-23.6, $p < 0.0001$).
Karlsson S. et al. 2008 [84].	Prospective cohort study (Finnsepsis study)	247 adult patients (59.3 years ±15.6 years) (mean ± standard deviation) with severe sepsis. 70 with bacteraemia.	Serum HMGB1 within 24 hours and 72 hours of study entry/Western blot relative quantification to pooled health volunteer serum (densitometry) and ELISA for randomly selected subgroup from 247 cases (HMGB1 ELISA Kit II (Shino-Test Corporation, Kanagawa, Japan))	10 healthy volunteers (median: 0.65 ng/ml, inter-quartile range: 0.51 to 1.0)	Hospital mortality: survivor's median (day 0) HMGB1 3.6 ng/ml (inter-quartile range: 1.9 to 6.5). Non-survivor's median (day 0) HMGB1 3.9 ng/ml (inter-quartile range: 2.1 to 8.7) $p = 0.17$ (Mann-Whitney *U*- test). Author's conclusion: Serum HMGB1 concentrations were elevated in patients with severe sepsis, but did not differ between survivors and non-survivors and did not predict hospital mortality.

Author/Year of publication	Study type	Patients	Variable measured/Assay(s)	Controls	Outcomes
Huang L.F. et al. 2011 [85].	Prospective cohort study	106 adult patients (age: 33.6 ± 4.3 years) (mean ± standard deviation) with > 30% total body surface area burn. 59 develop sepsis, 47 did not develop sepsis. (Baseline characteristics dissimilar: burn area and number of operations).	Serum HMGB1 at postburn days 1, 3, 7, 14 and 21 days (HMGB1 ELISA Kit II (Shino-Test Corporation, Kanagawa, Japan)).	25 healthy volunteers (17 men and 8 women, age 28.6 ± 6.2 years) (mean ± standard deviation)	For the sepsis versus non-sepsis group, there was a statistical significant increase on the day 7, 14, and 21 HMGB1 levels but no difference on the day 1 and 3 levels. For the survivor sepsis versus non-survival group, there was a statistical significant increase on the day 3, 7, 14, and 21 HMGB1 levels but no difference on the day 1 levels. No adjustments made for potential confounders (burn area and number of operations). Author's conclusion: Extensive burn injury could result in significantly increased HMGB1 levels, which appears to be associated with the development of sepsis and fatal outcome of major burns.

difficult. Earlier studies have used semi-quantitative method with western blotting due to a lack of readily available commercial ELISA kits [6, 82]. The concentration of serum HMGB1 in patients with severe sepsis when estimated by western blotting would be in higher range of tens of ng per ml (up to more than 100 ng per ml) while that by ELISA would be in the lower range of ones to tens of ng/ml (Table 3). This demonstrates intrinsic differences between the assays.

Although commercial ELISA kits are now available, they underestimate the total HMGB1 due to the blocking of epitopes secondary to HMGB1 propensity to form complexes. This prevents its recognition by capture and/or detection antibodies. To overcome this, semi-quantitative method using immuno-blotting (western blot detection) have been performed after denaturing sodium dodecyl sulphate polyacrylamide gel electrophoretic separation [50]. Recently, the use of perchloric acid to dissociate the HMGB1 complexes have been suggested during the ELISA detection [86]. This unmasking method has allowed detection of a much higher quantity of HMGB1 in the plasma of patients with septic shock as compared to non-perchloric acid ELISA. Given the enhancing effects that HMGB1 complexes have, measuring both the total and free HMGB1 may be helpful in understanding its role in sepsis.

Conclusion

Collectively, DAMPs are important mediators of sepsis. Among them, extracellular HMGB1 has one of the greatest potential as a therapeutic target due to its delayed release kinetics creating a clinically relevant timeframe for intervention and its independent key role in mediating lethality [6]. In addition, antagonism of HMGB1 is also able to prevent organ dysfunction in endotoxemic mice which is an important morbidity in severe sepsis (Table 2) [64] (Table 2).

Early experimental extra-corporeal blood cleansing device has already been shown to improve the survival in animal sepsis model through the targeted removal of PAMPs using magnetic nanobeads coated with an engineered human mannose-binding lectin (an endogenously occurring soluble PRR) [87]. However, the therapy was instituted very early targeting the early sepsis mediators. Similar depletion techniques but targeting late mediators such as HMGB1 instead would potentially offer ample response time for administration after diagnosis is made. Concurrently, improvements in quantification methods for HMGB1 including the ability to differentiate free and heterocomplex forms as well as its different redox variants will help us to understand its immunological role in severe sepsis such that in the future, more rational therapy can be instituted.

Acknowledgments

This work is supported by the Singapore National Research Foundation under its Clinician Scientist-Individual Research Grant-New Investigator grant and administered by the Singapore Ministry of Health's National Medical Research Council. In addition, Joo Guan Yeo is supported by the ExxonMobil research fellowship for clinician.

References

[1] Vincent, J.L., et al., International Study of the Prevalence and Outcomes of Infection in Intensive Care Units. *Jama-Journal of the American Medical Association*, 2009. 302(21): p. 2323-2329.

[2] Angus, D.C., et al., Epidemiology of severe sepsis in the United States: analysis of incidence, outcome, and associated costs of care. *Crit Care Med*, 2001. 29(7): p. 1303-10.

[3] Casey, L.C., R.A. Balk, and R.C. Bone, PLASMA CYTOKINE AND ENDOTOXIN LEVELS CORRELATE WITH SURVIVAL IN PATIENTS WITH THE SEPSIS SYNDROME. *Annals of Internal Medicine*, 1993. 119(8): p. 771-778.

[4] Fisher, C.J., et al., Treatment of septic shock with the tumor necrosis factor receptor:Fc fusion protein. *New England Journal of Medicine*, 1996. 334(26): p. 1697-1702.

[5] Fisher, C.J., et al., Recombinant human interleukin-1 receptor antagonist in the treatment of patients with sepsis syndrome - results from a randomized, double-blind, placebo-controlled trial. *Jama-Journal of the American Medical Association*, 1994. 271(23): p. 1836-1843.

[6] Wang, H.C., et al., HMG-1 as a late mediator of endotoxin lethality in mice. *Science*, 1999. 285(5425): p. 248-251.

[7] Bustin, M., Regulation of DNA-dependent activities by the functional motifs of the high-mobility-group chromosomal proteins. *Molecular and Cellular Biology*, 1999. 19(8): p. 5237-5246.
[8] Bianchi, M.E. and M. Beltrame, Upwardly mobile proteins. Workshop: the role of HMG proteins in chromatin structure, gene expression and neoplasia. *EMBO Rep.*, 2000. 1(2): p. 109-14.
[9] Janeway, C.A., Jr., The immune system evolved to discriminate infectious nonself from noninfectious self. *Immunol. Today*, 1992. 13(1): p. 11-6.
[10] Bianchi, M.E., DAMPs, PAMPs and alarmins: all we need to know about danger. *J. Leukoc. Biol*, 2007. 81(1): p. 1-5.
[11] Chen, G.Y. and G. Nunez, Sterile inflammation: sensing and reacting to damage. *Nature Reviews Immunology,* 2010. 10(12): p. 826-837.
[12] Andersson, U. and K.J. Tracey, HMGB1 is a therapeutic target for sterile inflammation and infection. *Annu. Rev. Immunol*, 2011. 29: p. 139-62.
[13] Lotze, M.T. and K.J. Tracey, High-mobility group box 1 protein (HMGB): Nuclear weapon in the immune arsenal. *Nature Reviews Immunology*, 2005. 5(4): p. 331-342.
[14] Medzhitov, R. and C. Janeway, Jr., Innate immunity. *N. Engl. J. Med.,* 2000. 343(5): p. 338-44.
[15] Lu, J.H., et al., Binding of the pentamer/hexamer forms of mannan-binding protein to zymosan activates the proenzyme C1r2C1s2 complex, of the classical pathway of complement, without involvement of C1q. *J. Immunol.*, 1990. 144(6): p. 2287-94.
[16] Lu, J., X. Wu, and B.K. Teh, The regulatory roles of C1q. *Immunobiology*, 2007. 212(4-5): p. 245-52.
[17] Lu, J., et al., Biosynthesis of human ficolin, an Escherichia coli-binding protein, by monocytes: comparison with the synthesis of two macrophage-specific proteins, C1q and the mannose receptor. *Immunolog*y, 1996. 89(2): p. 289-94.
[18] Epstein, J., et al., The collectins in innate immunity. *Curr. Opin. Immunol.*, 1996. 8(1): p. 29-35.
[19] Fraser, I.P., H. Koziel, and R.A. Ezekowitz, The serum mannose-binding protein and the macrophage mannose receptor are pattern recognition molecules that link innate and adaptive immunity. *Semin. Immunol.*, 1998. 10(5): p. 363-72.
[20] Takeda, K., T. Kaisho, and S. Akira, Toll-like receptors. *Annu. Rev. Immunol.,* 2003. 21: p. 335-76.

[21] Akira, S. and K. Takeda, Toll-like receptor signalling. *Nat. Rev. Immunol.,* 2004. 4(7): p. 499-511.
[22] Janeway, C.A., Jr. and R. Medzhitov, Innate immune recognition. *Annu. Rev. Immunol.,* 2002. 20: p. 197-216.
[23] Harris, H.E., U. Andersson, and D.S. Pisetsky, HMGB1: a multifunctional alarmin driving autoimmune and inflammatory disease. *Nat. Rev. Rheumatol.*, 2012. 8(4): p. 195-202.
[24] Yang, H. and K.J. Tracey, Targeting HMGB1 in inflammation. Biochimica *Et Biophysica Acta-Gene Regulatory Mechanisms*, 2010. 1799(1-2): p. 149-156.
[25] Andersson, U., et al., High mobility group 1 protein (HMG-1) stimulates proinflammatory cytokine synthesis in human monocytes. *J. Exp. Med.*, 2000. 192(4): p. 565-70.
[26] Bonaldi, T., et al., Monocytic cells hyperacetylate chromatin protein HMGB1 to redirect it towards secretion. *EMBO J.,* 2003. 22(20): p. 5551-60.
[27] Gardella, S., et al., The nuclear protein HMGB1 is secreted by monocytes via a non-classical, vesicle-mediated secretory pathway. *EMBO Rep.,* 2002. 3(10): p. 995-1001.
[28] Youn, J.H., et al., High mobility group box 1 protein binding to lipopolysaccharide facilitates transfer of lipopolysaccharide to CD14 and enhances lipopolysaccharide-mediated TNF-alpha production in human monocytes. *J. Immunol.*, 2008. 180(7): p. 5067-74.
[29] Lotze, M.T., et al., The grateful dead: damage-associated molecular pattern molecules and reduction/oxidation regulate immunity. *Immunol. Rev.*, 2007. 220: p. 60-81.
[30] Ito, I., J. Fukazawa, and M. Yoshida, Post-translational methylation of high mobility group box 1 (HMGB1) causes its cytoplasmic localization in neutrophils. *J. Biol. Chem.,* 2007. 282(22): p. 16336-44.
[31] Dumitriu, I.E., et al., Release of high mobility group box 1 by dendritic cells controls T cell activation via the receptor for advanced glycation end products. *J. Immunol.*, 2005. 174(12): p. 7506-15.
[32] Dumitriu, I.E., et al., Requirement of HMGB1 and RAGE for the maturation of human plasmacytoid dendritic cells. *Eur. J. Immunol.*, 2005. 35(7): p. 2184-90.
[33] Semino, C., et al., NK/iDC interaction results in IL-18 secretion by DCs at the synaptic cleft followed by NK cell activation and release of the DC maturation factor HMGB1. *Blood,* 2005. 106(2): p. 609-16.

[34] Scaffidi, P., T. Misteli, and M.E. Bianchi, Release of chromatin protein HMGB1 by necrotic cells triggers inflammation. *Nature,* 2002. 418(6894): p. 191-195.

[35] Bell, C.W., et al., The extracellular release of HMGB1 during apoptotic cell death. *Am. J. Physiol. Cell. Physiol.*, 2006. 291(6): p. C1318-25.

[36] Youn, J.H. and J.S. Shin, Nucleocytoplasmic shuttling of HMGB1 is regulated by phosphorylation that redirects it toward secretion. *J. Immunol.,* 2006. 177(11): p. 7889-97.

[37] Venereau, E., et al., Mutually exclusive redox forms of HMGB1 promote cell recruitment or proinflammatory cytokine release. *J. Exp. Med.,* 2012. 209(9): p. 1519-28.

[38] Yang, H., et al., Redox modification of cysteine residues regulates the cytokine activity of high mobility group box-1 (HMGB1). *Mol. Med*., 2012. 18(1): p. 250-9.

[39] Schiraldi, M., et al., HMGB1 promotes recruitment of inflammatory cells to damaged tissues by forming a complex with CXCL12 and signaling via CXCR4. *J. Exp. Med.*, 2012. 209(3): p. 551-63.

[40] Li, J.H., et al., Structural basis for the proinflammatory cytokine activity of high mobility group box 1. *Molecular Medicine*, 2003. 9(1-2): p. 37-45.

[41] Yang, H.A., et al., A critical cysteine is required for HMGB1 binding to Toll-like receptor 4 and activation of macrophage cytokine release. *Proceedings of the National Academy of Sciences of the United States of America*, 2010. 107(26): p. 11942-11947.

[42] Kazama, H., et al., Induction of immunological tolerance by apoptotic cells requires caspase-dependent oxidation of high-mobility group box-1 protein. *Immunity,* 2008. 29(1): p. 21-32.

[43] Diener, K.R., et al., The multifunctional alarmin HMGB1 with roles in the pathophysiology of sepsis and cancer. *Immunol. Cell Biol.*, 2013. 91(7): p. 443-50.

[44] Hreggvidsdottir, H.S., et al., The alarmin HMGB1 acts in synergy with endogenous and exogenous danger signals to promote inflammation. *J. Leukoc. Biol.,* 2009. 86(3): p. 655-62.

[45] Ivanov, S., et al., A novel role for HMGB1 in TLR9-mediated inflammatory responses to CpG-DNA. *Blood*, 2007. 110(6): p. 1970-81.

[46] Tian, J., et al., Toll-like receptor 9-dependent activation by DNA-containing immune complexes is mediated by HMGB1 and RAGE. *Nature Immunology*, 2007. 8(5): p. 487-496.

[47] Urbonaviciute, V., et al., Induction of inflammatory and immune responses by HMGB1-nucleosome complexes: implications for the pathogenesis of SLE. *J. Exp. Med.,* 2008. 205(13): p. 3007-18.
[48] Cully, M., Connective tissue diseases: HMGB1 helps elicit anti-dsDNA antibody production in SLE. *Nat. Rev. Rheumatol.*, 2013. 9(6): p. 321.
[49] Wen, Z., et al., Autoantibody induction by DNA-containing immune complexes requires HMGB1 with the TLR2/microRNA-155 pathway. *J. Immunol.,* 2013. 190(11): p. 5411-22.
[50] Urbonaviciute, V., et al., Factors masking HMGB1 in human serum and plasma. *J. Leukoc. Biol.*, 2007. 81(1): p. 67-74.
[51] Kokkola, R., et al., RAGE is the major receptor for the proinflammatory activity of HMGB1 in rodent macrophages. *Scand. J. Immunol.*, 2005. 61(1): p. 1-9.
[52] Yu, M., et al., HMGB1 signals through toll-like receptor (TLR) 4 and TLR2. *Shock,* 2006. 26(2): p. 174-179.
[53] Park, J.S., et al., High mobility group box 1 protein interacts with multiple Toll-like receptors. *American Journal of Physiology-Cell Physiology,* 2006. 290(3): p. C917-C924.
[54] Park, J.S., et al., Involvement of toll-like receptors 2 and 4 in cellular activation by high mobility group box 1 protein. *J. Biol. Chem.*, 2004. 279(9): p. 7370-7.
[55] Chen, G.Y., et al., CD24 and Siglec-10 selectively repress tissue damage-induced immune responses. *Science,* 2009. 323(5922): p. 1722-5.
[56] Hreggvidsdottir, H.S., et al., High mobility group box protein 1 (HMGB1)-partner molecule complexes enhance cytokine production by signaling through the partner molecule receptor. *Mol. Med.*, 2012. 18: p. 224-30.
[57] Huttunen, H.J., et al., Receptor for advanced glycation end products-binding COOH-terminal motif of amphoterin inhibits invasive migration and metastasis. *Cancer Res.*, 2002. 62(16): p. 4805-11.
[58] Chuah, Y.K., et al., Receptor for Advanced Glycation End Products and Its Involvement in Inflammatory Diseases. *Int. J. Inflam.*, 2013. 2013: p. 403460.
[59] Youn, J.H., et al., Identification of lipopolysaccharide-binding peptide regions within HMGB1 and their effects on subclinical endotoxemia in a mouse model. *Eur. J. Immunol.*, 2011. 41(9): p. 2753-62.

[60] Calogero, S., et al., The lack of chromosomal protein Hmg1 does not disrupt cell growth but causes lethal hypoglycaemia in newborn mice. *Nat. Genet.*, 1999. 22(3): p. 276-80.

[61] Ye, C., et al., Human macrophage and dendritic cell-specific silencing of high-mobility group protein B1 ameliorates sepsis in a humanized mouse model. *Proc. Natl. Acad. Sci. U S A,* 2012. 109(51): p. 21052-7.

[62] Yanai, H., et al., Conditional ablation of HMGB1 in mice reveals its protective function against endotoxemia and bacterial infection. *Proc. Natl. Acad. Sci. U S A*, 2013. 110(51): p. 20699-704.

[63] Abeyama, K., et al., The N-terminal domain of thrombomodulin sequesters high-mobility group-B1 protein, a novel antiinflammatory mechanism. *J. Clin. Invest.*, 2005. 115(5): p. 1267-74.

[64] Yang, H., et al., Reversing established sepsis with antagonists of endogenous high-mobility group box 1. *Proceedings of the National Academy of Sciences of the United States of America*, 2004. 101(1): p. 296-301.

[65] Wang, H., et al., Cholinergic agonists inhibit HMGB1 release and improve survival in experimental sepsis. *Nature Medicine*, 2004. 10(11): p. 1216-1221.

[66] Qin, S., et al., Role of HMGB1 in apoptosis-mediated sepsis lethality. *J. Exp. Med*, 2006. 203(7): p. 1637-42.

[67] Suda, K., et al., Anti-high-mobility group box chromosomal protein 1 antibodies improve survival of rats with sepsis. *World J. Surg.*, 2006. 30(9): p. 1755-62.

[68] Lutterloh, E.C., et al., Inhibition of the RAGE products increases survival in experimental models of severe sepsis and systemic infection. *Crit. Care*, 2007. 11(6): p. R122.

[69] Pan, P., et al., Low-dose cisplatin administration in murine cecal ligation and puncture prevents the systemic release of HMGB1 and attenuates lethality. *J. Leukoc. Biol.*, 2009. 86(3): p. 625-32.

[70] Chorny, A., et al., Ghrelin protects against experimental sepsis by inhibiting high-mobility group box 1 release and by killing bacteria. *J. Immunol.*, 2008. 180(12): p. 8369-77.

[71] Chorny, A. and M. Delgado, Neuropeptides rescue mice from lethal sepsis by down-regulating secretion of the late-acting inflammatory mediator high mobility group box 1. *Am. J. Pathol.*, 2008. 172(5): p. 1297-307.

[72] Hussein, M.H., et al., Effect of hemoperfusion using polymyxin B-immobilized fiber on IL-6, HMGB-1, and IFN gamma in a neonatal sepsis model. *Pediatr. Res.,* 2005. 58(2): p. 309-14.

[73] Ulloa, L., et al., Ethyl pyruvate prevents lethality in mice with established lethal sepsis and systemic inflammation. *Proc. Natl. Acad. Sci. U S A,* 2002. 99(19): p. 12351-6.

[74] Buras, J.A., B. Holzmann, and M. Sitkovsky, Animal models of sepsis: setting the stage. *Nat. Rev. Drug. Discov*., 2005. 4(10): p. 854-65.

[75] Faust, S.N., R.S. Heyderman, and M. Levin, Coagulation in severe sepsis: a central role for thrombomodulin and activated protein C. *Crit. Care Med.,* 2001. 29(7 Suppl): p. S62-7; discussion S67-8.

[76] Yamakawa, K., et al., Treatment effects of recombinant human soluble thrombomodulin in patients with severe sepsis: a historical control study. *Crit. Care,* 2011. 15(3): p. R123.

[77] Vincent, J.L., et al., A randomized, double-blind, placebo-controlled, Phase 2b study to evaluate the safety and efficacy of recombinant human soluble thrombomodulin, ART-123, in patients with sepsis and suspected disseminated intravascular coagulation. *Crit. Care Med.*, 2013. 41(9): p. 2069-79.

[78] Ohndorf, U.M., et al., Basis for recognition of cisplatin-modified DNA by high-mobility-group proteins. Nature, 1999. 399(6737): p. 708-12.

[79] Whitehead, K.A., R. Langer, and D.G. Anderson, Knocking down barriers: advances in siRNA delivery. *Nature Reviews Drug Discovery*, 2009. 8(2): p. 129-138.

[80] Barnay-Verdier, S., et al., Emergence of autoantibodies to HMGB1 is associated with survival in patients with septic shock. *Intensive Care Med,* 2011.

[81] Sakamoto, Y., et al., Relationship between effect of polymyxin B-immobilized fiber and high-mobility group box-1 protein in septic shock patients. *ASAIO J.,* 2007. 53(3): p. 324-8.

[82] Sunden-Cullberg, J., et al., Persistent elevation of high mobility group box-1 protein (HMGB1) in patients with severe sepsis and septic shock. *Crit. Care Med.,* 2005. 33(3): p. 564-73.

[83] Gibot, S., et al., High-mobility group box 1 protein plasma concentrations during septic shock. *Intensive Care Med.*, 2007. 33(8): p. 1347-53.

[84] Karlsson, S., et al., HMGB1 as a predictor of organ dysfunction and outcome in patients with severe sepsis. *Intensive Care Med.*, 2008. 34(6): p. 1046-53.

[85] Huang, L.F., et al., Association of high mobility group box-1 protein levels with sepsis and outcome of severely burned patients. *Cytokine*, 2011. 53(1): p. 29-34.
[86] Barnay-Verdier, S., et al., PCA-ELISA: a sensitive method to quantify free and masked forms of HMGB1. *Cytokine,* 2011. 55(1): p. 4-7.
[87] Kang, J.H., et al., An extracorporeal blood-cleansing device for sepsis therapy. *Nat. Med.*, 2014. 20(10): p. 1211-6.

Index

B

C

J

K

L

M

N

O

P

R

S

S

T